HARD CHOICES

HARD CHOICES

HEALTH CARE AT WHAT COST?

**DONALD DRAKE, SUSAN FITZGERALD,
and MARK JAFFE**
of The Philadelphia Inquirer

Andrews and McMeel
A Universal Press Syndicate Company
Kansas City

ABB 9930

Designed by Barrie Maguire

Library of Congress Cataloging-in-Publication Data

Drake, Donald, 1935–
    Hard choices : health care at what cost? / Donald Drake, Susan
FitzGerald, and Mark Jaffe of the Philadelphia Inquirer.
        p.   cm.
    ISBN 0-8362-8041-5 : $5.95
    1. Medical care—United States. 2. Medical care—Canada.
3. Medical care—Germany. 4. Medical, State—Canada.
5. Medical, State—Germany. 6. Medical policy—United States.
I. FitzGerald, Susan. II. Jaffe, Mark. III. Title.
RA395.A3D73   1993
362.1—dc20   93-32947
                                                                          CIP

CONTENTS

INTRODUCTION

I t became clear with the 1991 election of Senator Harris Wofford, Democrat of Pennsylvania, that people were worried about health care. They worried about paying their bills and losing their health insurance. They worried about becoming sick and going broke. Wofford's repeated calls to overhaul the nation's medical system caught the public's attention and proved crucial to his victory.

When the presidential campaign took off in early 1992, health-care reform was once again a key issue. Candidates talked about a need for change, though what shape that change should take was fuzzy at best.

In a series of casual meetings early in 1992, a group of reporters and editors working for *The Philadelphia Inquirer*'s SMASH desk (Science, Medicine, Aging and Social Health) began to brainstorm ways to bring home to readers the issue of health-care reform.

We had all read the news reports filled with comments from economists and health-policy experts, detailing the intricacies of medical systems in other countries. What we hadn't read was what it was like to be a patient in these other systems. What would it be like to be treated by a doctor or admitted to a hospital in a country where health care is guaranteed for all and spending is limited?

To answer that question, we decided to travel to two countries whose medical systems were being held up as worthwhile models—Canada and Germany—and compare what we saw there with what we saw in the United States. We selected three hospitals, one in suburban Philadelphia, one in Toronto, and one in Munich, as the basis for our reporting.

To get a patient's view of things, we divided our inquiry into four phases: A day in the life of a hospital in each country; a day with three family doctors; the experience of birth in each country; and heart bypass surgery. We spent hours in operating rooms, sat quietly in the corner of delivery rooms, and followed doctors from early morning to late at night. *Inquirer* photographer Akira Suwa was with us every step of the way, complementing our written words with his sensitive and insightful photographs.

What resulted was a five-part series that was published in *The Philadelphia Inquirer.* This book is a product of that work.

There were many friends and colleagues at the *Inquirer* who helped us along the way, and we want to thank them.

SMASH desk editors Charles Layton and Dotty Brown nurtured our ideas, bolstered our enthusiasm, and provided the fine editing touch for which they are known.

Executive Editor Jim Naughton served as an early critic and counselor and helped get this project moving. Metropolitan Editor Butch Ward provided key resources that enabled us to execute the project and was willing to let his reporters travel far afield.

Much of the credit for the newsroom atmosphere that enabled both reporters and editors to look beyond the obvious daily story and probe for new ways to approach the news goes to the *Inquirer*'s editor, Maxwell E.P. King.

Throughout the many months we worked on the series, our colleague Huntly Collins served as a sounding board and ad-hoc editor. Joe Daley of the *Inquirer* library staff worked wonders with data bases and dug up all sorts of useful information.

Kirk Montgomery, Barbara Binik, and Ray White of the *Inquirer* art department turned mind-boggling statistics into understandable graphics. Rhonda Dickey copyedited the series, with backup help from Richard Barron. Bob Filarsky designed the pages.

This project would not have been possible without the tireless cooperation of patients and staff members at each of the hospitals where we spent time. We particularly want to thank Richard Wells of Lankenau Hospital, Ruth Lewkowicz of North York General Hospital, and Dr. Dieter Eichenlaub of Schwabing Hospital, who enabled us to get complete access to their hospitals. The Munich leg of our trip was made easier thanks to Helmut Karcher, Marion von Gwinner, and Christine Wieselsberger, who served not only as translators but as guides to their beautiful city.

—Donald C. Drake
—Susan FitzGerald
—Mark Jaffe

CHAPTER 1

TO BE A PATIENT: A VIEW FROM THE UNITED STATES, CANADA, AND GERMANY

  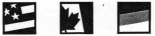

Jacqui Deabenderfer was anxious as she and her husband, Steve, drove up from their home in Cape May, New Jersey, to Lankenau Hospital in Wynnewood, Pennsylvania. In a few hours, the twenty-six-year-old mother was scheduled for surgery to remove precancerous cells from her cervix. She knew it was silly, but she was terrified she might never wake up from the anesthesia.

Steve tried his best to comfort her, but he had his own concerns. He kept worrying about the money—hoping he could work out an affordable payment plan with the hospital. The Deabenderfers had no health insurance.

With Jacqui so frightened, Steve, twenty-eight, kept his fears to himself as they drove to the hospital. Besides, he figured, they could worry about the money later. For now, he just wanted his wife to get the best care possible. But it wouldn't be that easy.

Arriving at Lankenau, they crossed the carpeted lobby and gave their name to a clerk, who handed Jacqui an admission slip. The box marked "no insurance" had been checked. You have to go to the financial office, the clerk said.

■

The Deabenderfers were about to suffer a frustrating but quintessential American experience—a financial confrontation with the nation's medical system.

More and more hard-working Americans now face this obstacle when they're sick and need care. As companies pull back on medical benefits, and as more people lose their coverage, the nation is searching for ways to reform its system.

One of Bill Clinton's first acts as president was to appoint a task force headed by his wife, Hillary Rodham Clinton, to quickly deliver a comprehensive national health-care plan that would totally rethink how Americans get their medical care. Driving the president's concern was this disturbing fact: America spends more on medical care than any other industrialized country—70 percent more per person than Germany. Yet there's no evidence we get better care.

Other advanced countries manage to insure everybody, fairly and equally. The United States leaves one in seven people completely uninsured and many more insured for just a portion of their needs. Those other countries do what we cannot because, over the years, they've made hard choices—choices we are only now, reluctantly, starting to consider. They put limits on spending, and make those limits stick. They use expensive technology more sparingly than we do, and more efficiently. They've streamlined administrative costs, so they spend a fraction of what we do on paperwork. And they limit doctors' fees.

The two countries that draw the most attention for their efforts are Canada and Germany. They are very different. Canada's system is tax-supported and government-run. Germany's relies on insurance funds that are highly regulated, but private. The two together demonstrate that there's more than one way to keep costs down while delivering good health care for all—an important thought as America debates these issues.

What the Three Countries Cover

Canada spends $1,915 per capita and covers everyone for:
- Hospitalization.
- Doctor visits.
- Rehabilitation therapy.
- Most dental work.
- Prescription drugs for the poor, not for others.
- Most lab tests.

Germany spends $1,659 per capita and covers everyone for:
- Hospitalization, with $8-per-day co-payments.
- Doctor visits.
- Most dental work.
- Prescription drugs, with co-payments up to $4.90.
- Lab tests and eye glasses.

United States spends $2,867 per capita and:
- Leaves 15 percent of population uninsured.
- Sets no coverage standards; many who are insured have spotty coverage.

All figures from 1991

Just by roaming the halls of these countries' hospitals, you can see the strengths and weaknesses of their systems. These become obvious in the individual dramas that unfold in the treatment rooms, wards, and corridors.

In Canada and Germany, you'll sometimes see patients waiting for hours to get care. But you will never hear a German or Canadian being asked the unsettling question, "How do you plan to pay?"

You will see patients who face delays in getting the high technology that's so abundant in this country. But those same patients will tell you that theirs is the best health-care system in the world.

You will see emergency rooms in Germany that are virtually empty because doctors are out roaming the city in the middle of the night, making house calls.

You will see Canadian hospitals that save money by sharing high-technology equipment linked by telephone lines. And, in the United States, hospitals engaged in wasteful duplication, racing to see which can amass the most, the latest, the fanciest, and the costliest technology.

You will see how Canada and Germany have chosen to make trade-offs to keep costs down—but not the kind of "rationing" that many Americans fear.

And you'll see how the United States makes trade-offs, too—trade-offs the other two countries have refused to make because of the burdens they would place on patients.

This book uses three comparable hospitals for close-up observation—North York General Hospital in Toronto, Schwabing Hospital in Munich, and Lankenau Hospital on the outskirts of Philadelphia. Each is considered among the best community hospitals in its city—a place people go for superior care. And the way those people are treated tells much about how that nation's health-care system really works.

Spend twenty-four hours in each of these very different places, and see for yourself.

6:30 A.M.: Emergency Room, North York General

Dawn was breaking, and Joan Evans, a woman in a white, flowered nightgown, had been lying in Toronto's busiest emergency room for more than twelve hours. She had injured her head in a fall and was waiting to be admitted. But since all of North York General's beds were filled, Evans had to bide her time until a room opened up.

She wasn't alone. The emergency room was packed. All but two of the nineteen curtained examining cubicles were filled. Four more patients lay in beds along the wall. And seven others, Joan Evans among them, were in a cluster of beds behind the nurses' station, where they tried to sleep as best they could.

Many of the patients had already been examined, and ten were deemed sick enough for admission. But most wouldn't get a room until late morning or early afternoon, and a few would have to wait until the next day. This happens a lot at North York, which is forced to strike a delicate balance nearly every day between patient demand and available resources.

North York is a private, nonprofit hospital, but its funding comes from tax dollars. Under Canada's system, the government in each province decides every year how much it will spend on health care, and it parcels the money out to all hospitals and doctors through negotiations. Every hospital gets a "global budget"—a fixed amount for the year. The hospital has to make do with that—and give care to everyone who shows up.

While health care is a big-ticket item in the budgets of each of Canada's ten provinces—in Ontario it consumes one-third of all revenues, more than education, transportation, or housing—demands for care and the costs of providing it continue to rise. With only so much money to work with, North York and other hospitals have to set priorities and make hard choices. In 1992, North York closed a forty-bed ward to save money, though it put a strain on the emergency room.

Despite some inconveniences, surveys show that most Canadians think highly of their medical system. They see the occasional waiting as a price they have to pay for the comprehensive care they are guaranteed.

This was certainly true of the patients in North York's emergency room this morning. Many were dozing. Some lay propped on pillows, reading magazines or books. One woman was knitting. An American reporter wandered from bed to bed, interviewing patients about the Canadian health-care system and provoking some lively discussion. When the reporter came near Joan Evans—even before a question was out of his mouth—she blurted out: "We don't have socialized medicine. We have social responsibility."

Although she'd been waiting in the ER since 5:30 the

evening before, Evans said she was here by choice. Under Canada's system, she could go to any hospital she chose. And many of the others probably had beds, because on a given day, Toronto has one thousand empty hospital beds. But Evans liked North York. She'd been here before, and this was the first time she'd had to wait.

8 A.M.: Ward XO, Schwabing

Josefa Hägel woke up wondering whether she'd finally get to leave the hospital today. For nearly two weeks, the ninety-two-year-old Munich woman had been tested and monitored for heart trouble, but the doctors had found nothing. They'd told her she might get to go home if the final test results were normal.

Hägel had been rushed here with the classic signs of a heart attack—chest pain and shortness of breath—after her doctor had called "Bed Central" to find out which hospital in Munich had a free bed. It turned out to be Schwabing Hospital—the oldest of Munich's four municipal hospitals, with long, linoleum-floored hallways, well-worn furnishings, and some rooms that must share toilets.

Hägel's room was spare but clean. It had two early-model hospital beds and was furnished with a couple of plastic chairs, a print of the city of Essen in medieval times, and a small table with a vase of flowers. She had neither a television nor a telephone, but she did have a private toilet.

Hägel is a sprightly woman whose gray hair is matched by gray, sparkling eyes. You couldn't find a much better expert on German health care—at least from the patient's viewpoint—than she is.

Germany has the world's oldest health-care system, started in 1883 by Otto von Bismarck. The system was only seventeen years old when Hägel was born into it.

Over her lifetime, she has been in the hospital for the birth of her children, pneumonia, abdominal surgery, and several other operations. And she's been covered all her life by the same insurance company, the Allgemeine Orts-krankenkasse, or AOK.

Virtually all Germans are covered through a network of these nonprofit insurers, called "sickness funds." There are nearly twelve hundred, of which AOK is the largest. The sickness funds get their money through payroll contributions averaging 12.5 percent of wages, with employees and employers splitting the payment. The funds cover hospitalization, doctor visits, pharmaceuticals, dental work, and physical therapy. The government pays premiums for the unemployed. Premiums for retirees are paid by their pension funds. The only people not in the funds are the destitute, who are covered by welfare agencies, and the affluent, who can opt out of the system by purchasing private insurance.

Each year, the sickness funds negotiate rates with doctors and hospitals. The government acts as referee, mandating what has to be covered and setting spending targets. Since only so much money is available, the sickness funds, hospitals, and doctors act as counterbalancing forces in dividing it up.

Of the several Munich hospitals that Hägel has been in, she was especially impressed by Bogenhausen, the city's newest municipal hospital. "It was very good, so modern," she said. But, she added, "Schwabing is fine. . . . The doctors take the time to sit down and talk to you and always ask about your life," she said, "whether you've been married, if you have children."

If Hägel went home today, she would leave with a bill of $112, representing her copayment of $8 a day for fourteen days. The rest of her bill—about $4,100—would be paid by AOK.

Never has Hägel worried about health-care costs. For

nearly a century, through two world wars, AOK has paid the bills. "It always covered what was necessary," she said. "I've never had a problem. I never thought about it."

9 A.M.: Finance Office, Lankenau

When Jacqui and Steve Deabenderfer entered Lankenau's financial services office, they were greeted by Patti Yost, a dark-haired woman with black reading glasses. Her office was decorated with cheerful posters and a lamp with a bright yellow shade.

Yost is one of Lankenau's two credit representatives, who interview patients to make sure the hospital's bills will be paid. Seeing the "no insurance" box checked off on the admission slip, Yost asked Jacqui and Steve if they could make a deposit for Jacqui's surgery, a laser procedure to get rid of the dangerous cells on her cervix.

This was the second time the young, middle-class couple had come face-to-face with a stark reality of the United States medical system: Unless it's an emergency, nobody gets medical care until payment is guaranteed. Three years earlier, while Jacqui was in labor with their son, Drew, at a New Jersey hospital, a labor room nurse told Steve to go to the financial office to arrange for time payments for the impending birth. It ended up costing $2,800, and they've been paying monthly installments of $40 or more ever since. They won't have it all paid until after Drew's fourth birthday.

Yes, Steve told Patti Yost, they were prepared to make a deposit of $400. Yost told them that wasn't enough. The hospital bill might be about $3,000. She wanted a 50 percent down payment.

Steve Deabenderfer was stunned. He earned $29,500 a year as a salesman for a food-supplies company. His wife was a homemaker who did some part-time waitressing.

Steve knew they could never manage the kind of terms Yost was talking about.

Steve continued to bargain, but the best he could do was talk Yost down to a $1,000 deposit, with the balance due in a month. That was still an awful lot for them to pay. Yost suggested the couple might qualify for state Medicaid funds if they went back to New Jersey, where they lived.

They explained that they had come to Lankenau because they thought it offered the best chance of preserving Jacqui's fertility. A New Jersey doctor had told Jacqui that the surgical treatment required to remove her precancerous cells could affect her chances of having a second child. The couple wanted very much to have another baby.

Jacqui's eyes began to fill. Yost could see that she and Steve were very disturbed. The credit representative stood up. She said she would be back in a moment.

9:15 A.M.: Day Surgery, Lankenau

Esther DeLeo, a seventy-seven-year-old woman with twelve grandchildren, was about to get her second cataract operation at Lankenau. DeLeo loved the hospital, loved her ophthalmologist, and loved that she could have her operation in the morning and be home in time for the afternoon radio talk shows.

Lankenau also liked DeLeo. She was exactly what the hospital looks for in a patient. She had not one but two insurance policies—her basic Medicare coverage and supplemental Blue Cross and Blue Shield, which paid for drugs, semiprivate room, and other niceties not provided by the federal plan. Clearly, DeLeo's bill would be paid—a crucial consideration for any U.S. hospital.

The United States has one of the few free-market medical systems left in the industrialized world. It also has the most inflationary system of all, with doctors and hospitals

The Three Hospitals

Lankenau Hospital

Philadelphia

Lankenau, with carpeted halls and color-coordinated wards, looks more like a hotel than a place where pain, sickness, and death are confronted. The community hospital in suburban Wynnewood draws patients from both city and suburbs. It is packed with medical technology and offers many sophisticated procedures, rivaling large university hospitals.

Total beds	475
Admissions	16,630
Patient days per year	128,176
Avg. length of stay	7.6 days
Nurses per bed	1.9
Occupancy rate	74%
Operating budget	$153 million

North York General Hospital

Toronto

From its new emergency room to its radiology department that runs 12 hours a day, North York General is one of the busiest hospitals in Toronto. Its lobby is packed with patients and visitors sipping gourmet coffees served from a green-canopied cart. The suburban community hospital leaves most high-tech services to the downtown teaching hospitals.

Total beds	473
Admissions	21,292
Patient days per year	158,805
Avg. length of stay	7.8 days
Nurses per bed	1.3
Occupancy rate	88%
Operating budget	$79 million

Schwabing Hospital

Munich

Built at the turn of the century, Schwabing is a sprawling campus of stucco structures connected by long, windowed hallways. One of Munich's four municipal hospitals, it provides no-frills, quality care attracting rich and poor alike. It is a major center for diabetes, children's surgery, and cardiology, but lacks high-tech services like MRIs and heart surgery.

Total beds	1,372
Admissions	43,491
Patient days per year	404,936
Avg. length of stay	9.2 days
Nurses per bed	0.8
Occupancy rate	85%
Operating budget	$196* million

*Includes doctors' salaries

Figures from 1992.

able to provide whatever services they want, usually with the assurance that they'll be paid.

The best way for a hospital such as Lankenau to survive, and give quality care, is to attract all the well-insured patients it can. It does this by assembling under one roof an amazing array of medical services, and incorporating fancy flourishes, from valet parking to carpeted wards and recessed lighting.

This day, DeLeo's encounter with the American medical system would be markedly different from the Deabenderfers'. Unlike them, all her papers were in order. So she was fully entitled to what the system does best—provide technologically advanced care, quickly and competently.

"This is a consumer-driven system," says Elizabeth Avery, Lankenau's president. "The consumer still has a lot of choice." If DeLeo hadn't liked her first cataract operation at Lankenau, there were probably ten other hospitals within easy driving distance offering the same surgery.

She was sure her surgery would, once again, go well, and that she'd be home for her afternoon talk shows. And that's exactly how it turned out.

9:20 A.M.: Billing Office, Lankenau

As the Deabenderfers' frustrating drama unfolded in financial services, the neighboring billing office was a blur of activity. There, dozens of hospital staffers were chasing after hundreds of pending hospital bills.

Sitting in cubicles with computer terminals and reams of files, these employees tracked bills both old and new, some stretching back two years. In all, fifty-three people would spend this day at Lankenau making sure the hospital got the money it needs to operate.

This was no easy task, considering how many ways there are in the United States to pay medical bills. Medicaid, run by the states, covers the poor. The federal Medicare program pays for the elderly. And about 1,200 commercial insurance companies cover people through their jobs or individually. It's such a complicated, time-consuming business that Lankenau's finance section is larger than its departments of pediatrics, obstetrics, or radiology.

"Hello, this is Lankenau Hospital," one of the billing representatives said. "I would like to check the status of a claim. We've heard nothing."

Angela O'Donnell, who handles commercial insurance claims for Lankenau, was calling Travelers Insurance Company in Augusta, Georgia, about a $2,498 bill. She gave the patient's name and claim number, waited a bit, and then was told that the company would get back to her.

This was how O'Donnell spent every working day, phoning insurance companies all over the country. This day, she would speak to Met Life, Central Reserve Life, Pioneer Life, Aetna, and the Guardian. And on her desk were files involving Crum & Foster, Benefit Concepts, Keystone Health Plan, Prudential, Weaver Associates, PruCare, Provident, Beacon Corporation, Benefit Services, Cigna, Planned Services, and the Major League Baseball Players Benefit Plan.

Every plan offered a different type of coverage. One had a $1,500 deductible, another had a $300 deductible plus a $150 deductible for every hospital admission, and another had a $125 deductible and then 80 percent coverage until the patient spent another $400, after which full coverage kicked in.

North York General in Toronto doesn't have to spend its time or money badgering insurance companies. Because its budget is almost totally funded by the government at the start of every year, it can make do with a dozen people in its billing office. The only things patients pay for are extras, such as TVs and semiprivate rooms. (Sixty-five percent of Canadians have supplemental insurance that pays for those rooms.)

The German billing system is equally hassle-free, and Schwabing—with three times as many beds as Lankenau—needs only eighteen people to do the job. When a patient is discharged from Schwabing, the hospital calculates the bill by multiplying the number of days in the hospital by a fixed daily rate determined by the type of illness. (The base rate is about $344.) This one bill covers every aspect of treatment—doctors, lab work, and any other medical tests. The bill is sent to the sickness fund, which pays the hospital in two to six weeks. Simple as that.

German hospitals spend eight cents on the dollar for administration and paperwork. Canadian hospitals spend nine cents. American hospitals, according to the Harvard School of Public Health, spend about twenty cents.

American insurance companies also spend a lot on administration—12 percent of every premium dollar, according to Harvard. A German sickness fund such as AOK spends only about 5 percent on administration, while Canada, with its government-run system, spends just 1 percent.

An hour after her phone call to Travelers, Angela O'Donnell got a call back. Travelers had decided it would pay $1,900. This was $598 less than Lankenau's bill. The patient would have to pay the difference. "This always gets patients angry," O'Donnell said. "They get a bill months after they leave the hospital and blame us."

9:30 A.M.: Finance Office, Lankenau

"Let's go home and let them do whatever they want to me in New Jersey," Jacqui Deabenderfer said as she and her husband waited for Patti Yost to return. Steve felt terrible. He remembered how, when they first decided to come to Lankenau, he had told his wife they'd find a way to pay for her surgery "no matter what."

The Deabenderfers had come to this impasse because they believed they had the right to choose their doctor and hospital. But like most American workers, the Deabenderfers actually had little say in what medical insurance they would buy, or what it would cover. That was determined by the company Steve worked for. When, for cost-cutting reasons, his last company switched from Blue Cross to a health maintenance organization (HMO), the couple's choice of doctors and hospitals was restricted to those that participated in the HMO.

Jacqui's care at Lankenau wouldn't have been covered by the HMO because Lankenau wasn't a participant in the plan. So rather than buying into the HMO while Steve was between jobs, the couple decided to drop insurance coverage altogether and apply the money they'd save on premiums to Jacqui's operation. In doing that, the couple joined the thirty-seven million Americans who have no health insurance at all.

The Deabenderfers were reviewing their options when Yost returned with her boss, finance services manager Joseph Elsasser. From Elsasser's viewpoint, the problem wasn't just Jacqui's $3,000 laser surgery. What if something went wrong? Serious complications could run her bill into tens of thousands of dollars, which Elsasser knew the couple could never pay.

So accepting Jacqui was a financial risk for Lankenau. Still, Elsasser told the couple that if they were willing to pay the $1,000 deposit Lankenau had asked for, the hospital would work out an arrangement for the rest.

Steve Deabenderfer took out his checkbook. He had a balance of $1,150, mostly severance money from the job he had just left. He wouldn't be paid by his new employer for another week.

Elsasser couldn't say exactly what kind of payment terms could be worked out. The hospital would have to review the couple's financial situation. But nothing could be done until Steve made a satisfactory deposit.

Deabenderfer wrote out the check and handed it to Elsasser. The financial services manager gave Deabenderfer some forms to fill out. The couple would have to provide pay stubs, tax returns, a list of debts, expenses, and other data. If, once the forms were returned, Elsasser decided to give the couple a break on their bill, he would have to recommend that to his boss, June Landis, the business manager. She, in turn, would have to recommend it to her boss, Robert Kauffman, assistant vice president for finance, who has the power to act on matters involving $10,000 or less.

More costly proposals also require the approval of the vice president for finance, Anthony Acchione. But since the Deabenderfers' case was a small one—probably involving a risk of less than $2,000—it had to go through only two levels of approval.

Elsasser didn't explain all this. He just said that the hospital would get back to the couple in a week or two. That settled, he told the Deabenderfers that Jacqui could go upstairs for surgery.

11:15 A.M.: Chemotherapy Clinic, North York General

Armand Jelilyan was sitting in an armchair in the chemotherapy clinic with an intravenous line in his arm. Though Canada's limits on technology can cause some waiting, most patients, like Jelilyan, get fast, efficient treatment.

Five months earlier, the thirty-three-year-old accountant had gone to his family doctor with "a cough that just wouldn't go away." The doctor detected a couple of lumps on the left side of his neck and immediately sent him to have an X ray and an ultrasound.

The very next day, he was sent to a cancer specialist at North York General, who performed a biopsy. A second biopsy was done the following week. He also had a CAT scan, a bone marrow test, and an injectable dye scan to search for cancer. Within three weeks, he had been diagnosed as having Hodgkin's disease.

A week later, he began chemotherapy at North York as an outpatient. Through it all, Jelilyan has continued his job and has even been able to play some hockey. "Although," he said, "I've had to cut back a bit."

After six months of treatment, Jelilyan was scheduled for a month of radiation therapy at the Bayview Regional Cancer Centre at nearby Sunnybrook Health Science Centre. Jelilyan faced no delay in booking his treatments. But in Ontario, cancer patients have had to wait anywhere from a few weeks to several months, depending on the type of radiation therapy they needed. Such periodic backups are part and parcel of a system that tries to walk the line between too few and too many resources. To relieve the backlog, some patients were referred to hospitals as far as 225 miles away. The government paid all their expenses for travel and lodging.

Waiting lists aren't the only problem. North York General's global budget from the government does not include money to operate the chemotherapy clinic where Jelilyan was getting his treatment. But the hospital decided to operate the clinic anyway.

"We just felt that it was a service our community needed," said Carole Oliver, a hospital vice president. To finance the clinic's operation, the hospital depends on about $120,000 a year in community fund raising.

North York General and the government disagree on other budget matters as well. For example, because the hospital has one of the busiest maternity wards in Toronto, it operates a neonatal intensive-care unit. Yet, the government hasn't designated the hospital a neonatal care center, nor has it added extra money to the institution's budget. So North York has to juggle its priorities.

"We at least have the option of shifting resources," said Murray MacKenzie, the hospital's president. "Maybe someone will have to wait longer for plastic surgery . . . or perhaps we have to close some beds."

Still, it is a frustrating exercise for MacKenzie. In the 1992 fiscal year, the hospital received $66.1 million from the government and augmented that with an additional $13.2 million from such miscellaneous sources as parking charges and fees for semiprivate rooms. It still ran a deficit for the year of about $213,000.

"I don't have sufficient resources at the moment to run North York General at the level of quality I would like to," MacKenzie said.

1:30 P.M.: Hospital Corridors, Schwabing

Dressed in a navy robe with white and red flowers, and pushing an intravenous pole on wheels, Lieselotte Fischer, sixty-one, took a mid-afternoon stroll down the hallway of her ward at Schwabing Hospital. Then she returned to her room and settled back into bed.

Fischer, who had worked in the shoe business before her retirement, had been operated on for intestinal cancer two months earlier at Neuperlach, a municipal hospital on the other side of Munich. Her family doctor recommended Neuperlach because it specializes in that type of surgery. She underwent two cycles of chemotherapy there but had to switch to Schwabing for radiation because Schwabing is the municipal hospital that specializes in that.

After her radiation and drug treatments, Fischer would have to move to yet a third hospital, for her *Kur* or "cure."

This would be a rehabilitation hospital, where she'd undertake an exercise program and learn how to live a healthier life.

In Germany, the local hospital doesn't try to be all things to all patients the way U.S. hospitals do. Instead, as Fischer's case shows, specialized services are confined to certain hospitals. This is cheaper and more efficient. Often, a critically ill heart-surgery patient will go to the intensive care unit of one hospital, stay there until the eve of surgery, then be transferred to another hospital for the operation, and then, twenty-four hours later, come back to the original hospital to recover.

Such moving about is unheard of in the United States. But in Germany, both the government and market forces militate against American-style duplication of services. Public and nonprofit hospitals must negotiate with the state government for capital improvement funds. And in Bavaria, where Munich is located, the money is disbursed in such a way that technology and specialized facilities are sprinkled across the state, according to Dr. Gerhard Knorr, a top official in the Bavarian Ministry of Labor, Family, and Social Welfare. "We try to have a regional plan . . . ," Knorr said, "which balances the interests of the politicians, the doctors, the hospitals. Everyone wants something else."

Knorr acknowledged that "if you live in a rural area you may have to drive 120 miles" for procedures like cardiac catheterization, magnetic resonance imaging (MRI) scans, and lithotripsy for crushing kidney stones.

Private doctors are free to set up private hospitals and buy just about any technology they want, using private funds. But to make it pay, they must negotiate contracts with the sickness funds, which are wary of too much technology because it drives up premium rates. Even the regional physicians' association tries to discourage some big-ticket items, for fear of diluting doctor fees. There's only so much money to go around.

In Canada, the duplication of services so common in America does not happen as often, either, because hospitals are trying to live within their global budgets. MacKenzie is fond of saying that in Canada, medical resources are not "rationed," as many Americans suspect, but that resources are "rationalized."

For example, North York General and Sunnybrook hospitals, which serve roughly the same area, avoid duplicating specialized services. Sunnybrook offers heart and brain surgery; North York doesn't. North York has an obstetrics ward; Sunnybrook doesn't. North York does geriatric psychiatry, and Sunnybrook does adolescent psychiatry. MacKenzie said he thinks rationalization is one of the keys to survival for Canadian hospitals, and "the only way to assure centers of excellence."

3 P.M.: Day Surgery, Lankenau

Jacqui Deabenderfer was lying in a bed in day surgery. Her operation had gone well. In a twenty-minute procedure, surgeon Norman Rosenblum had used a laser to vaporize the precancerous cells on Jacqui's cervix.

Steve was with her in the recovery room, and they were talking about when it might be all right to start trying for their second baby. They knew it would depend on the results of Jacqui's postsurgical Pap smear. A negative smear would mean the surgery had gotten rid of all the dangerous cells.

Suddenly, the two of them were struck by the same thought. "We better get out of here," they said almost in unison, "before they charge us for another day."

Jacqui, feeling stronger, quickly got dressed. An hour later they were back on the highway, headed home. Exhausted, Jacqui dozed in the seat beside her husband, and Steve was alone with his thoughts about money. He hoped

Lankenau would agree to either reduce its bill or set up a long-term payment plan the couple could live with.

But that was up to Lankenau. There was nothing the Deabenderfers could do but wait for the hospital to decide.

3:15 P.M.: Radiology Department, North York General

Raziel Gershater, North York's chief of radiology, was sitting in a darkened room, surrounded by glowing video screens and humming computers. Three miles away, at Sunnybrook Hospital, Charles Glover, a junior high school geography teacher with a bad back, was being wheeled into an MRI room.

The images of Glover's back from the MRI machine would be transmitted over telephone lines to the video screens at North York, where Gershater would analyze them. Even though the MRI is at Sunnybrook, North York owns a piece of it and gets to use it two days a week. This keeps costs down.

As far as Gershater is concerned, two days is simply not enough time. "If we have an urgent case, we can't get it in until the next week," he complained.

New technology is exciting for doctors but a problem for the government, which has to pay the bills. A single MRI machine can cost anywhere from $1.5 million to $3 million. "The government has a low-tech mind-set," Gershater said. "They want to stay away from the stuff because it costs a lot. They delay introduction of high technology as long as they can."

Toronto, with a population of 3.7 million, had five MRI machines in 1993. In Philadelphia, the Hospital of the University of Pennsylvania alone had that many. All told, the Philadelphia metropolitan area, with 4.9 million people, had sixty-three MRI machines.

Doctors in Toronto order MRI scans much more sparingly than do doctors in Philadelphia. Canadian patients can wait months for their name to come up on the list. In Canada, Gershater said, "You have the absurd situation where doctors feel that they should only use this tool in a dire, life-or-death situation."

Not everyone agrees. Gordon Cheung, director of the MRI unit at Sunnybrook, said he thinks everyone in Canada who needs an MRI scan gets one. But he also wishes more time were available on the machine for research.

Canada limits more than just MRIs. Per capita, the nation has one-eighth as many radiation therapy units as the United States, one-fifth as many lithotriptors for treating kidney stones, and one-third as many cardiac catheterization units.

If technology were solely in the hands of the German government, the story might be the same there. But unlike Canada, Germany allows more room for private enterprise. Schwabing's radiology department has no MRI machines at all, but even so, it takes only two or three days for a nonemergency patient to get an MRI. That's because hospitals can turn to private physicians. They, not the hospitals, own and operate most of the MRI machines. Munich, with 1.3 million people, has ten MRIs, twice as many as Toronto—eight in doctors' offices and two at university hospitals.

Overall, Canada has 0.5 MRI machines for every one million people, Germany has 0.9, and the United States has 3.7 MRIs.

3:45 P.M.: Nurses' Station, Lankenau

Registered nurse Carolyn Vozzo got off the elevator, walked to the nurses' station and started going through patients' charts.

But she wasn't there to take care of patients. Vozzo is a

utilization review nurse, one of five that Lankenau employs to make sure no patient stays longer than necessary. Instead of a thermometer and stethoscope, Vozzo's only tool is a rolled-up bunch of bright orange stickers.

Checking an average of forty charts a day, Vozzo will slap a sticker on the chart of any patient who no longer seems sick enough to need hospital care. Then it's up to the doctor to discharge the patient or explain why that can't be done. The ultimate penalty for ignoring the orange labels is loss of hospital admitting privileges, but it has never come to that.

Vozzo perused the chart of an elderly male patient getting intravenous antibiotics for an infection and shots of painkillers for low back pain. No need for a sticker yet. She would check back in three days.

She scrutinized the chart of an eighty-three-year-old woman who had been admitted through the emergency room with pneumonia. The care seemed appropriate, but no one had started planning for her discharge. This was potentially dangerous to the hospital. If no one was available outside the hospital to take care of the woman, Lankenau might have to keep her longer—and be stuck for the cost.

Moving patients out of hospitals expeditiously is the single major effort the U.S. health-care system has made to cut costs. Medicare, the nation's insurance program for the elderly, started the initiative in 1984. Instead of reimbursing patients based on the number of days they were in the hospital, Medicare started paying a flat price for each treatment—so much for a gall bladder operation, so much for an appendectomy. Now some insurance companies, also anxious to cut costs, have adopted the same payment method, known as DRGs (diagnostic related groups). Some have hired their own utilization review staff.

DRGs force hospitals to be more efficient. If a hospital gets a patient out faster than expected, it makes more money. If the patient lingers, it loses money.

Patients are feeling the impact. People are discharged who aren't sick enough to stay in the hospital, but are too sick to be on their own. They put a strain on friends and relatives, and create a demand for home health-care workers and nursing homes.

In Canada, patients spend an average of fourteen days in the hospital. In Germany, it's seventeen days. In the United States, the average is nine days. Lankenau's average is less than that. In three years, it has cut its average length of stay from nine days to seven-and-a-half.

4 P.M.: Medical Ward, Lankenau

It was nearly time for Irene Goldfeld, an eighty-four-year-old woman with a broken ankle, to be discharged from the hospital. Goldfeld broke her ankle stomping on a bug.

"I only remember I was in my living room, the lights were on bright, and I saw a bug—a big, black bug—and it wouldn't move," Goldfeld said. "This one seemed to be looking at me; it was like it was waiting for me. I stepped on it and fell."

Her hospital stay had gone well, but now that she was close to being discharged, she had no place to go. Her right foot was in a cast, and her doctor had said she couldn't put weight on it for ten weeks.

"I'm in a bad predicament because I live alone," she had told a hospital social worker, Caroline Wexler, earlier in the day. "I have no one to help me. What am I going to do in an apartment by myself?"

Wexler had come to talk to Goldfeld about her discharge. Though the social worker had a full schedule, she took a lot of time with the woman, holding her hand and giving her a Kleenex for her crying sniffles.

Lankenau employs eleven social workers, most of whom,

like Wexler, spend their time figuring out how patients' medical needs will be met once they leave the hospital. The move to shorter hospital stays has made this task all the more critical.

"When people ask what social workers do, I used to say they help people cope with illness," Wexler said. "Now the primary reason hospitals employ social workers is to make sure people have safe discharge plans . . . and that doesn't mean calling the taxicab."

Wexler told Goldfeld that Medicare would pay for her time in the hospital, but once she left, getting help wouldn't be easy. Medicare would pay for aides to come to her home to give very limited nursing care. It might even pay for a couple of weeks in a rehab facility, but probably nothing longer than that.

"I called Bryn Mawr Rehab this morning," Wexler told Goldfeld, referring to an institution a few miles away. "I said, 'Is there any chance of Medicare coverage for a fractured ankle?' They said, 'No, not usually.'"

Wexler said she was still waiting to hear whether Haverford Nursing and Rehabilitation Center, another nearby institution, would take Goldfeld.

Evelyn Shapiro, Goldfeld's sister, who was visiting, said she couldn't see why her sister was being left in such a predicament. "I'm seventy-five. I can't take care of her," Shapiro told the social worker. "She doesn't have any money. What's a senior citizen to do?"

Both sisters were crying now.

"You get frightened and you get scared," Shapiro said.

4 P.M.: Medical Ward, Schwabing

 Ward X0 was full—all thirty-four beds were occupied—but head nurse Gisela Eiwanger had only two nursing assistants this afternoon to help her. A comparable ward in the United States might have ten staffers.

"There's always a shortage of nurses," said Eiwanger, who was dressed in typical German nursing garb—a white chemise, black leotards, and Earth sandals. "A lot of the people working on the ward just have a year of training. It's a big problem. You really can't give all the care that should be given."

Doctors agree. When a Harvard Medical School study asked German physicians what was the country's biggest medical problem, 77 percent cited the shortage of nurses.

In prestige and salary, nursing ranks much lower in Germany than in Canada or the United States. "Normally, women who are trained as a nurse only spend four years on the job and then do something else," Eiwanger said.

A thirty-year-old nurse at Schwabing makes at most $475 a week. A German schoolteacher makes $543. A nurse at Lankenau makes about $770. The average base salary for an R.N. at North York is $726.

U.S. hospitals have much higher staffing ratios than hospitals in Germany. In 1987, the last year for which international data are available, the United States averaged 3 staffers per bed and Germany averaged 1.3. Canada's average was 2.5.

Of course, German hospitals need fewer nurses because they have a smaller concentration of acutely ill patients than American hospitals. This, again, is because Americans try to discharge people as soon as they pass the acute phase of care.

Still, by any standard, Germany is short of nurses. For Eiwanger, the shortage means having to cut lots of little corners. It means getting help from interns and residents in taking lab samples and giving injections. It means letting the patients who can walk bus their own food trays from a serving cart in the hall.

And it means giving patients all their medication for the

day in one delivery. The nurse leaves a plastic tray in the room with compartments marked "morning," "midday," "afternoon," and "night," and depends on the patients to take their pills on time. That saves the nurse three trips later in the day.

With patients suffering pneumonia, pancreatitis, stroke, Alzheimer's, and a host of other ailments, Eiwanger is always on the run. "Everyone is stretched thin," she said.

5:30 P.M.: Surgical Ward, North York General

Ana Rico, sixty-seven, who had just undergone a three-hour knee operation, was snoring under an oxygen mask. In the next bed was a woman eating broccoli. The strong smell permeated the room. Across from Rico, another patient was talking loudly on the phone, updating someone on her medical condition. The fourth bed in the room belonged to a woman who was arguing with a nurse about her medications.

But Rico snored away, oblivious to it all—oblivious, too, to the victory she had just won. Finally, after six months, she had gotten her long-awaited surgery.

Canadians actually get more of some types of surgery— gall bladders, for instance—than patients in the United States. But they have to wait longer for highly specialized procedures such as knee or hip replacements.

Rico's doctor, orthopedic surgeon Robert Brock, said his patients usually wait six months for those operations. While they wait, he said, "they hobble around with pain, they take anti-inflammatory drugs, they take painkillers, they sit around at home."

Brock is limited by the availability of operating-room time, which is carefully doled out among all kinds of surgeons at North York. At some university centers in Toronto, he said, orthopedic surgeons are booking patients more than a year in advance.

Researchers who have studied waiting lists in Canada say that some delays are inevitable in a system that tries to make maximum use of resources. "You can't have a system that runs on tight resources, that has efficiencies pushed by capped budgets, without occasionally having logjams," said C. David Naylor, a Sunnybrook researcher. But in some areas—and orthopedic surgery is one—Canada clearly needs more facilities, he said.

In the United States, hip or knee replacements can be scheduled within weeks. In Germany, patients wait about three months.

As Ana Rico slept, her daughter, Martha Escobar, waited outside in the hallway. She was relieved that her mother had come through the knee surgery with no problems. Escobar said her mother's osteoarthritis had gotten so bad in the previous year that she couldn't even get on a bus to go shopping. Now, with her artificial left knee, she should have little trouble getting around.

"She couldn't wait until the day of the operation," Escobar said.

8:45 P.M.: Sleep Clinic, Lankenau

In Lankenau's Sleep Disorder Center, a technician was wiring twenty electrodes to the head, torso, arms, and legs of Edward Sciubba, in preparation for the night. Plopped on Sciubba's chest was a control box about the size of a TV remote channel changer.

Sciubba, fifty, a securities trader, suffered from a dangerous and exhausting condition called sleep apnea. Hundreds of times a night he would stop breathing.

For the second night in a row, machinery would monitor his brain waves, eye movements, heart rate, breathing, and muscle tone. A small microphone placed just in front of his nose would even record his snoring. Sciubba would be one of three patients evaluated this night in the sleep center.

The center is one of several boutique-like clinics at Lankenau that reflect an expensive trend in American medicine—the packaging and marketing of special medical services to attract patients who can pay.

Popping up at hospitals all around the country are headache clinics, chest-pain clinics, executive-health clinics, and clinics for the "mature woman." Because American medicine is seen as a product to be promoted and sold, hospitals are always looking for new ways to package their services, to lure the customers. So the department of radiology begets the breast clinic. And the department of orthopedic surgery takes on new life as the sports medicine clinic.

Lankenau's sports medicine clinic looks remarkably like a Center City health club, with its mauve and maroon decor, Nautilus equipment, and monogrammed T-shirts. Its breast diagnostic center is even more elaborate. It has a color scheme of teal and rose with flecks of lilac, and is filled with women who wear dusty-rose examining robes as they wait to have mammograms. "The ladies comment all the time on the decor," said Linda Farinella, the clinic supervisor. "They love it."

Not surprising, considering that Lankenau hired an office design firm and spent $431,000 outfitting the clinic. "There is a tremendous competition among hospitals these days," said Lankenau vice president John Marcy. "Competition for shrinking reimbursement dollars."

As part of its marketing strategy, Lankenau, like most American hospitals, tries to offer as wide a range of tests, procedures, and services as possible, lest a patient have to go elsewhere and never return. It's akin to one-stop shopping. "You've got to remember," said Leonard Karp, vice president of the Delaware Valley Hospital Council, "we are the society that brought the grocery store into the gas station."

While Germany and Canada tend toward efficient, no-frills care, they occasionally indulge in American-style extravagance to attract patients. A breast-imaging clinic near North York General is almost as plush as Lankenau's. And Munich has some posh private hospitals, such as Privat-klinik Josephinum, a 130-bed facility with carpeting, wood paneling, and brass trimming around the front door.

The big difference between the luxury medical services in the United States and those in Germany and Canada is that only the well-insured are targeted in the United States. In the other countries, everyone is welcome because everyone is well insured.

9:20 P.M.: Emergency Room, Lankenau

The late-night collection of minor complaints had started drifting into Lankenau's emergency room. A man with a sprained ankle. A woman with a dislocated shoulder. A man with painful hemorrhoids. A woman with a cut finger. A five-year-old girl with an upset stomach.

They came here because they had no place else to go. Either they didn't have a family doctor or their doctor's office was closed. Although Lankenau's emergency room is state-of-the-art, with specially equipped rooms for treating heart attacks, chemical burns, and trauma, most of the people who come here have far more mundane needs.

This is not the most economical way to give routine care. Lankenau's typical charge for an emergency visit is $147. This is four times the cost of a visit to a doctor's office. But for many Americans, especially the poor who can't afford a family physician, the emergency room *is* the family physician. A study for Congress by the General Accounting Office found that nearly half the people treated in hospital emergency rooms do not need urgent care. The report noted that many have nowhere else to go.

10 P.M.: Emergency Room, Schwabing

As night descended on Munich, the emergency room at Schwabing was dead quiet. A lone nurse in the medical section was reading a newspaper while a cleaning woman mopped the floor in the hallway. It had been quiet like this for hours.

This was not unusual. For one thing, real emergencies are sent immediately to intensive care or surgery. And people with minor problems don't turn up in Germany's emergency rooms; they call their family doctor. But another reason the emergency room was empty was Thomas-Michael Grasser, who this evening was out riding around in a radio taxi with his doctor's bag.

Every night, four doctors cruise Munich, making house calls. People who can't get hold of their family doctors for a problem can call a number at the regional physicians' association in downtown Munich. The association set up the taxi system partly to keep nonemergencies out of the hospital, and partly to bolster the income of primary doctors. But in the end, it helps save money for the whole German health system.

This night, three hundred people would call the office, including the parents of a child with an asthma attack who wanted help, several people with infections and sore throats seeking advice, and a worried man with chest pain.

One call took Grasser to an apartment building in a working-class neighborhood. Lugging a sixteen-pound metal valise containing his medical instruments and drugs, Grasser jumped from the taxi and galloped up two flights of stairs.

"The quicker you go, the more you do," he explained.

The patient turned out to be two-year-old Taygun Aksan, who was running a fever. As soon as he saw Grasser, he began to cry. Using his best bedside manner and a borrowed teaspoon as a tongue depressor, the doctor examined the boy, took his temperature, listened to his chest, and looked into his throat and ears.

Grasser concluded that the boy had tonsillitis. He pulled from his bag an antibiotic powder and mixed it with water, producing an orange-colored drink. Taygun drank it reluctantly. His father asked for a prescription, which Grasser gave, along with the advice that if the fever wasn't down by morning the family should contact their regular doctor.

Grasser wrote down the necessary information to bill the family's sickness fund and was on his way. The fund would pay him $56 for this visit—ten times more than a daytime office visit costs.

"This kind of service is very expensive," he said. "But it's not big medicine."

And, it's a lot cheaper than treating a patient in a hospital emergency room.

None of these numbers mattered, though, to the working-class parents who were worried about their sick child. The house call, like all other medical care in Germany, was covered by their sickness fund.

Postscript

Jacqui and Steve Deabenderfer got the good news from Lankenau three weeks after returning home. Lankenau said it would not charge the couple any more than the $1,000 they'd already put down as a deposit. The hospital would write off the rest as part of the more than $2 million in charity care it provides each year. The couple would still have to pay the physicians' bills—$372 for the anesthesiologist, $365 for the pathologist, and $900 for the surgeon.

Three months after Jacqui's surgery, the health insurance provided by Steve's new job took effect. One month later, Jacqui became pregnant.

CHAPTER 2

A DAY IN THE LIFE
OF THREE DOCTORS

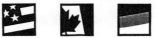

It was a little after seven A.M. when Ervin Fleishman walked into the hospital room of one of his longtime patients. The eighty-three-year-old woman was lying quietly as he sat down on the edge of her bed. The day before, she had come to his office for a regular checkup, complaining of indigestion and shortness of breath. "She's not a complainer, so when she complains, I listen," Fleishman said.

He gave her an electrocardiogram, saw menacing changes in the readout, and quickly admitted her to Lankenau Hospital. This morning she would have cardiac catheterization—a procedure to take pictures of her heart.

Holding her hand, he explained what would happen: "Dr. Sawin is going to do a catheterization. It is not going to hurt. . . . There will be a lot of equipment. . . . There will be a needle in the groin and when they inject the dye you may feel it. The table may be a little hard."

"You'll be there?" the woman asked.

"I'll be there, if they need me. Don't worry."

"Then I'll go home?"

"You're not ready to go home," Fleishman said softly. "We'll get you home."

■

Although they did not realize it, Fleishman and his patient were about to go on a turbulent ride through the American health-care system. It is a ride Fleishman knows too well. For while the system can offer the most sophisticated medicine—cardiac catheterization, CAT scans, and open-heart surgery—virtually on demand, it also can leave patients, families, and doctors confused, exasperated, and angry.

Fleishman is a primary-care physician practicing on the front lines of American medicine. He is the first and most enduring contact many patients have with the system. But America's health care market is dominated by specialists, making it a difficult place to practice basic medicine.

The story is very different in countries such as Canada and Germany, which have radically different health-care systems. In those countries, primary care—the brand of medicine dispensed by the old-fashioned family doctor—plays a more central role.

In Germany, Katherine Neubach practices in the modest Munich suburb of Neuaubing, where virtually everyone belongs to one of the country's nonprofit health insurance funds. Germany requires that the family doctor be the first stop for any medical complaint. "The goal," Neubach explains, "is for someone to be responsible for the patient."

Virginia Robinson is a physician in Canada, where the government pays for everyone's health care and also administers the system. There, as in Germany, the majority of community doctors are generalists. And Canada's Royal College of Physicians and Surgeons has decreed that specialists function mainly as "consultants" to the primary-care doctors.

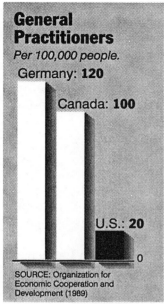

General Practitioners

Per 100,000 people.

Germany: **120**

Canada: **100**

U.S.: **20**

0

SOURCE: Organization for Economic Cooperation and Development (1989)

The Philadelphia Inquirer

Robinson has a family practice in upper-middle-class North Toronto. She has a long-standing relationship with many of her patients, having brought them into the world and cared for them and their families. Her patients can go to a specialist whenever they want, but the system strongly encourages them to check first with their family doctor.

In the United States, only thirty percent of doctors offer primary care, and even that group is split among family practitioners, general practitioners, pediatricians, gynecologists, and internists such as Fleishman.

"Our system has become fragmented," said Fleishman. That fragmentation sometimes results in patients being treated as ailments rather than people and, in Fleishman's view, "leads to poor communications and misunderstandings."

It also leads to an expensive brand of medicine. Studies have shown that specialists rely more on expensive tests, drugs, and hospitalization than family physicians and general practitioners do.

Neither Robinson in Canada nor Neubach in Germany has as ready access to high-tech medicine as Fleishman does. And neither makes as much money as Fleishman. In Canada and Germany, doctors' salaries have been a major target in efforts to hold down costs. Still, surveys by the Harvard School of Public Health have found that doctors and patients alike in Canada and Germany are far more satisfied with their systems than Americans are with theirs.

Robinson, Neubach, and Fleishman are all in their for-
ties, and all are experienced primary-care physicians. Each
is a private entrepreneur with a practice of about 2,500
patients—patients who freely chose them and could switch
if they were dissatisfied.

Yet their practices are very different. Spending a day
with each reveals how different it is to be a physician—and
to be treated by one—in each country.

An American Doctor's Day

 After leaving the elderly woman, Fleishman continued on his rounds of five other patients he had at
Lankenau.

Just about all Fleishman's admissions are to Lankenau.
Part of this is convenience—his offices are in the building
next door. But part of it is that the hospital, in an effort to
capture paying patients, requires him to send the large
majority of his admissions there. Failure to do so might
result in his loss of admitting privileges.

The last patient on his hospital rounds, however, was
one both he and Lankenau very much wanted out the
front door. She was a fifty-year-old woman who had come
to Fleishman's office a week before, barely able to walk
and complaining of chest pains. Fleishman quickly admitted her. Only then did he see her medical history. She had
twelve similar admissions. Twelve false alarms.

Still, he did a lung scan and an echocardiogram. Con-
vinced that there was no problem, Fleishman moved to
discharge the woman. But she insisted she was ill and
asked for a second opinion. A cardiologist at the hospital
suggested a stress thalium test. Fleishman argued that
the test was unnecessary. "That's OK," the woman told
Fleishman. "That's what they told my mother. She didn't

need the test, and she went home and keeled over and died."

The cardiologist did the test—a $531 charge. It was negative. Fleishman suggested the woman see a psychologist. She refused.

Then she told Fleishman, "It's got to be my ulcer, that's what they told me in the past." He was sure it wasn't an ulcer, and this morning he was determined to discharge her.

He walked to the nurses' station and pulled the woman's file. It had a bright orange sticker—like a parking ticket—slapped across the front. The hospital's utilization review nurse, who searches for cases where excessive care may have been given, had tagged the file. In her opinion, this was a case the insurance company might refuse to pay for. "Boy, they are getting me for everything," Fleishman said.

He usually considers utilization review's second-guessing "a slap in the face." "Sometimes you get so frustrated you feel like saying, 'Come take care of my patient. If you've got a better solution, be my guest.'" But there was no dispute here. The woman's discharge was overdue.

Fleishman entered the woman's room. She was sedated. A gastroenterologist, without Fleishman's knowledge, had just "scoped" her—placed a tube with a viewing device down her esophagus—to look for the ulcer that wasn't there. Fleishman was dismayed.

"Listen to me," he told his groggy patient. "I'm going to come back at the end of today . . . and maybe we will get you home today. . . . You've had a million dollars in tests here," he said.

"I'm glad someone else is paying for it," the woman replied.

■

The dominance in America of the cardiologist, the gastroenterologist, and other specialists is relatively new. In the early 1960s, half of all American doctors were generalists. But the growth in high-tech medicine, the promise of higher salaries, and the emphasis on specialties in medical schools has caused a tremendous growth in specialists. Between 1965 and 1990, the number of gastroenterologists jumped tenfold, orthopedic surgeons rose sevenfold, and the ranks of allergists tripled. The number of general practitioners declined 68 percent.

Perhaps it's not surprising that while family practitioners averaged $102,000 in net income in 1990, according to the American Medical Association, cardiologists made $262,200 and orthopedic surgeons netted $283,300. Average net income for internists, a group that includes both primary care doctors and specialists, was $152,500. Fleishman said he makes slightly less.

The rise in specialists has dramatically changed American medicine. "A patient who goes to a gastrointestinal specialist is more likely to be scoped," Fleishman said. "A cardiologist is more likely to call for studies. . . . I'm telling you that from being in everyday practice. That is what is going on. . . . The specialist isn't doing anything wrong. Patients are pushing for it and specialists are being extremely defensive, or maybe their reasons for studies are financial."

A study in *The Journal of the American Medical Association* in 1992 reported that when comparable patients were treated by internists and by specialists, the specialists tended to prescribe more hospitalization and more pharmaceuticals. Even Fleishman's patients constantly seek out specialists, to his consternation. "When a patient self-refers, the left hand doesn't know what the right hand is doing. . . . It is more costly. There is an increased risk and an increased chance of error," he said.

■

Fleishman returned to his office at 10:15 A.M. There were eight phone calls to return, and three patients waiting. An independent practitioner, Fleishman shares office space with another internist, Edward Laska. Between them, they employ four people—two for billing and two to handle appointments and records. This morning, Fleishman worked his way through cases of the flu, shingles, diabetes, hypertension, heart disease, and bronchitis, spending thirteen to twenty-one minutes with each patient.

His first patient was Terry Powers, a Keystone AAA executive with a bad case of bronchitis. Powers and his wife, Ann, both use Fleishman as their primary-care physician. "He is really first-class," Powers said. The couple see Fleishman once or twice a year. Their two children, however, go to a pediatrician and Ann also has a gynecologist. In addition, their son sees an allergist.

While Fleishman was doctoring, Margaret Lloyd was preparing bills. This day she would mail eighty-three bills to private patients, and file twenty-five bills with Medicare, the federally funded health insurance plan for the elderly. Lloyd sends out hundreds of individual bills each month. In some cases, it will be four months or more before they are paid.

"Your insurance company has rejected our bill," Lloyd informed one patient leaving the doctor's office. "That's why we sent the bill to you—twice."

There was a momentary silence. "They didn't pay? Who didn't pay?" the man asked.

"Prudential," Lloyd said.

"Oh, I'm not with them anymore. I'm with New Jersey Blue Cross," he replied.

"It would be nice if you'd let us know," Lloyd said with a diplomatic smile.

"Hey, I want to see you folks get paid, but it is not coming out of my pocket," the patient quipped.

On the counter, right where patients enter the office, is a sign. It is a sign found in many American doctors' offices. It is a sign of American medicine. It reads:

Payment Is Expected When Services Are Rendered Unless Other Arrangements are Made in Advance.

■

At 12:45 P.M., Fleishman finished with his last patient and hurried to Lankenau's cardiac catheterization lab. He wanted to see the pictures of the heart of the elderly woman who'd come in complaining of indigestion.

"This is a very tough situation," cardiologist Henry Sawin, Jr., told Fleishman. "The lady has a very strong heart and some very blocked arteries." He recommended bypass surgery.

Fleishman and Sawin went upstairs to talk with the family. "It is unstable angina. . . . It is a very angry area," Sawin said.

"Erv, what do you think?" the woman's daughter asked Fleishman.

"One of the things we look at is risk," Fleishman said. "We as doctors are trying to manage risk, and ironically the surgery is less risky in this case."

"How quickly can it be done?" the daughter asked.

The doctors contacted one of Lankenau's four cardiac surgeons. The answer: The surgery could be scheduled for the very next day.

After a quick sandwich, Fleishman was back in his office at 1:30 P.M. to deal with a serious case of poison ivy, a bad back, more cases of flu. By 4:30, he'd seen twenty-three patients and fielded twenty phone calls for the day. Late in the afternoon, he walked back to talk to his heart patient. Sitting on the edge of her bed, he explained the surgery.

A few minutes later, Fleishman was making an entry in the chart at the ward nursing station, when the woman's daughter came rushing out of the room. Her mother had suddenly become unresponsive. "Stay calm," Fleishman advised. He hurried back into the room and quickly examined the woman. He suspected a mini-stroke.

He phoned the neurologist on call and, while on hold, picked up a second phone and called the heart surgeon. The neurologist asked for Fleishman to arrange a CAT scan. Within two hours the scan would be done.

■

At 5:35 P.M., Fleishman returned to the room of the patient with the phantom heart condition and the imaginary ulcer.

"How are you feeling?" he asked cheerily.

"Terrible," she replied.

"Why do you feel terrible?" Fleishman asked. But without waiting for a detailed answer, he said, "I would like to get you home. . . . It is not your heart. There is no ulcer here. . . . As far as medicine goes, there is no reason to give you anything new." He finished the discharge form. "Now, I've discharged you," Fleishman pronounced. "Smile. Come on, you can do better than that."

The doctor returned to his office, finished a little paperwork, took another call. "Sam, as frustrating as it is for the moment, the best you can do is keep taking that cough medicine," he advised the caller.

At 6:25 P.M., almost twelve hours after coming to the hospital, Ervin Fleishman was out in the parking lot, a few feet from his Mercedes, when his beeper went off. He found a phone and called his answering service.

It was Henry Sawin, the cardiologist. He was very agitated. The elderly heart patient's family had heard from a nurse that the surgery had been canceled. Angry, they called Sawin, who knew nothing about it. Both Sawin and Fleishman suspected that the surgeon had pulled the plug on the surgery because of the suspected mini-stroke. "You're the case manager, do something," Sawin told Fleishman.

"I'll smooth it over," Fleishman said. "Let's let a little time pass and wait for the neurologist's report. . . . I'll take care of it."

It would not be until 10:30 that evening that everything would be sorted out. There was no stroke, and the surgery was done three days later. It was successful.

Fleishman headed back to his car. "You know, the irony of the situation is, every one of the doctors is going to file with Medicare, and Medicare may look at this case and it may decide only to pay the specialists, because it was clear what each of them did. "They may say to me, what did you do? This was a heart condition; it was the cardiologist's case."

A Canadian Doctor's Day

The day had just begun and Virginia Robinson was already late. She had dropped off her four-year-old daughter at nursery school, and now it was 9:05. Her first patient had been scheduled for nine.

Robinson hurried into the office, in a suburban medical building. The tranquil strains of Pachelbel's *Canon* were playing softly on the office tape deck. Toys and children's books were piled in one corner. Three patients were leafing through magazines. On the reception counter—about where Fleishman would have had his payment sign—was a photo of Robinson's two daughters in a silver frame.

All Robinson's patients are covered by the government-run Ontario Health Insurance Plan (OHIP), which pays for office visits, most lab tests, and hospitalization. "I never worry whether a patient can pay. It is never an issue," Robinson said. "Never."

Behind the desk was Diane Houston, the office manager. Houston works for Robinson and Dr. Janis Browne. Like Fleishman and Laska at Lankenau, Robinson and Browne share offices but have separate practices.

Unlike the two American doctors, they do not need four additional people to handle their office work. They manage with Houston and a registered nurse. The nurse handles all lab tests, shots, and telephone inquiries from patients. Houston manages appointments, files, and billing. She can do all this because the payment form is computerized, all bills go to the same payer—OHIP—and the office has every patient's OHIP insurance number in its computer data base.

New patients simply show their red-and-white plastic OHIP card and a valid address. That's all the doctor needs to get paid. It is a simple, equitable system, and both Robinson and her patients appreciate it.

"I've been in the States. I know what it is like," said Melinda Laventhol, who had come to Robinson's office to get an allergy shot for her six-year-old son, Joshua. "My son came down with scarlet fever when we were visiting relatives in New York. We were recommended to a specialist and we had to pay $110 up front before he would even see us," she said. "I appreciate the kind of system that we have. I know it is not the same everywhere else."

■

But it is a system under growing stress.

The problem is, Canada's free and open care has led to a health-care feeding frenzy. Between 1980 and 1990, Ontario's budget for health care tripled to about $12.8 billion. That translated to a 50 percent increase in health expenditures for every man, woman, and child in the province. Of course, the $1,400 per person that Ontario spent was almost 50 percent less than the average per capita in the United States.

Still, the government—which has to levy taxes to pay the bills—is trying to put the brakes on spending. One morning in 1992, Canadians picked up the newspaper to find Deputy Health Minister Michael Decter urging them to stay home and cope with their illnesses themselves.

"We don't want people rushing off to see their doctor at the first sniffle," Decter told the *Toronto Globe and Mail.*

"Most of the time, you can look after yourself. Have chicken soup."

Virginia Robinson agreed: "There are people who show up for every little thing."

But the government's solution is not chicken soup. It is rigorous control of technology and medical resources. That is why there is a $65,000 annual cap on the lab tests Robinson can order. It's also why 2,200 hospital beds have been closed in Toronto in recent years, and why the city has only one-tenth as many expensive magnetic resonance imaging (MRI) scanners as Philadelphia. The burden of managing these resources falls on hospitals and on physicians such as Robinson.

"The problem in our system is that we are broke and there is all this new technology . . . ," Robinson said. "People's expectations are very, very high. People know what's out there and want it and don't want to wait."

Every time Robinson has to send patients to the hospital, refer them to a specialist, or suggest they seek a particular treatment, she has to consider where and how they will receive the most expeditious care. For example, even though Robinson is on staff at North York General Hospital, she sends patients to any of a dozen hospitals—based on which one has beds available and which can best treat that patient's ailment.

It is not just doctors who wrestle with the problem. All Canadians are sensitive to it.

This day, Elizabeth Wilson, thirty, saw Robinson for a sore knee. The knee was easily treated, but Wilson was feeling the limits of her health-care system in other ways. She explained that during a regular checkup, Robinson had detected what appeared to be an ovarian cyst. Wilson was referred to a specialist who, as is sometimes the case in Canada, had a waiting list.

"I've been waiting the better part of two-and-a-half

months for laparoscopy," she said. "It's not the end of the world, but I'd like to know whether it is a cancer or a cyst."

Through the morning, Robinson dealt with cases ranging from bronchitis to high blood pressure to an infant's checkup. The classical music played on the tape deck, and the atmosphere was relaxed and friendly. But the undertone of concern is always there when Canadians discuss their health-care system.

"Ontario, as are the other provinces, is in a stressed financial situation," said Doreen Troutman-Smith, whose family of six is cared for by Robinson. "Each year it has become increasingly a worry what will happen if you get seriously sick."

Still, the Canadian system has done well by her. When her son fell off a swing in the summer of 1992 and broke his elbow, there was no waiting, no list, just quick, free care. "I was brought up in Boston . . . ," she said. "I would not want a system like the one in the United States. I think it is inconceivable that a basic level of health care simply is not provided."

■

One place where the Ontario government has sought to stem rising costs is physician salaries. In 1991, the government and physicians negotiated an agreement that if their collective billings exceeded a certain level they would return money to the government. In addition to this collective "payback," a cap of $320,000 a year was placed on individual doctors' incomes.

Robinson's net income is about $110,000. "My income has been static for the last five years," she said. "We got a 1 percent raise this year. It was big-time."

The trade-off for Robinson and other Canadian doctors is that payment is always prompt. One month, Robinson sent in 605 bills totaling $19,000. OHIP paid 598 of the

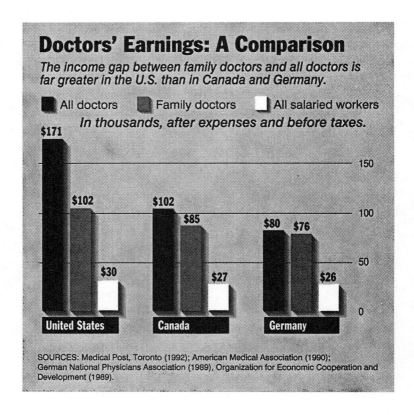

Doctors' Earnings: A Comparison

The income gap between family doctors and all doctors is far greater in the U.S. than in Canada and Germany.

■ All doctors   ■ Family doctors   ☐ All salaried workers

In thousands, after expenses and before taxes.

United States: $171, $102, $30
Canada: $102, $85, $27
Germany: $80, $76, $26

SOURCES: Medical Post, Toronto (1992); American Medical Association (1990); German National Physicians Association (1989), Organization for Economic Cooperation and Development (1989).

bills immediately, and questioned seven. "These claims errors are usually typos or clerical errors," Houston said.

Robinson augments her billings by making an annual pitch for a patient retainer. "We provide a family practice that is both caring and comprehensive," the retainer letter says. "We provide many diagnostic services right here in the office. . . . This kind of up-scale practice is expensive to run. Many services are not covered by OHIP. Should you not want to pay the retainer, we may have to bill for uninsured services." (These include renewing prescriptions and fielding phone calls.)

Robinson asks for $36 from individuals, $64 from families, and $18 from senior citizens and students. "I guess we get about $18,000 a year from the retainer letter," she said. A minority of Canadian doctors seek such retainers, but the idea is now being promoted by the Ontario Medical Association.

■

At one P.M., after a quick lunch at home with her husband, Robinson was back in her office.

Jane Stewart, an IBM executive, came in for a muscle spasm in her neck. In a six-year period starting in the late 1980s, she'd had a hysterectomy and a thyroid removal under the Canadian system without any problems. In both cases, the surgery was scheduled a couple of months in advance, and her additional Blue Cross coverage, part of IBM's fringe benefits, paid for extras such as a semiprivate room, phone, and television.

"My in-laws live in Phoenix, my stepfather has been in and out of the hospital over the last ten years. The care we've had here has been just as good but less expensive." She worries about the future, though. "We can't afford the system we have today. . . . I don't see how we can keep on."

A little after five P.M., Robinson had finished with the day's last patient. A total of thirty-three people had come to the office for complaints that included an irritable colon, an upper respiratory infection, anemia, vaginitis, and an ear infection. One teenage girl whose parents were in the middle of a messy divorce came in just to talk. Robinson saw eighteen patients, spending as much as a half hour with each.

She began to work through the afternoon's files, checking and organizing them before they went back to Diane Houston for billing. Then she phoned patients about lab results that had come back. One call was to a sixty-year-old woman suffering from arthritis. Her X rays showed the steady progress of the disease in her hips. "For the moment," Robinson said, "we can continue to manage this with anti-inflammatory drugs. But at some point down the road you are going to want the relief that an operation will give you."

The news made the patient anxious, because there have been waiting lists of up to six months for hip surgery. "Don't worry," Robinson assured. "When you need it . . . I will send you to the best surgeon and . . . to St. John's, the Cadillac of rehabilitation centers. . . . Don't worry, we will arrange everything."

A little after six, Robinson hurried home. "I have to get in close to six or I'll get hell from my nanny," she explained.

A German Doctor's Day

It was the middle of a very busy morning in Katherine Neubach's office when the call came in. One of her patients, a forty-year-old woman battling bowel cancer, was too sick to make it to chemotherapy. Neubach, a family doctor practicing in the Munich suburb of Neuaubing, had already seen twenty patients and would see a dozen more before lunch.

Still, the call from the woman's elderly mother concerned her. The patient had come to the office four months earlier with extreme weight loss. Neubach found the cancer. The woman was operated on within three weeks, but the disease had already spread to the lungs and liver.

The woman had begun chemotherapy with a nearby oncologist. But today, she was prostrate with diarrhea and nausea. "What happens [in cases like this] is that one morning you don't get up anymore . . . ," Neubach said. "I'm afraid this could be the beginning of the end."

In the United States or Canada, there isn't much a family doctor would or could do in a case like this—other than suggest the woman go to the nearest hospital. But after phoning the oncologist, Neubach determined that she could personally administer today's treatment—simple saline intravenous solutions. Neubach called the woman to say she would be there at noon. Before that, though, she had a full waiting room to deal with.

■

Neubach's day had begun at about 8:45 A.M. at her office in a small shopping complex. As a rule, German primary-care doctors don't give appointments except for lab tests and comprehensive physicals. Instead, they have "open hours"—first come, first served. And come they do. Between nine, when the office opened, and eleven A.M., when the hours "closed," there was a steady stream.

Patients first stopped at the reception desk. Christina Reidel, Neubach's "doctor's aide," would pull up their file on the computer. The screen showed the patient's name, address, age, insurance fund, and last two visits. Reidel is more than a receptionist. She is trained to give injections, draw blood for tests, and run the electrocardiograph machine.

This day, Neubach, with just Reidel's help, would see nearly twice as many patients as Fleishman sees in a normal day. In her Spartan private office, Neubach sat behind a glass-topped desk decorated with a small vase of red flowers and an ungainly yucca plant—a present from a patient. On her computer screen was the morning's waiting list. She would pull up a file on the screen, go to the door, call the patient, and return to the desk.

Sitting at the keyboard, she took notes while interviewing the patient and then conducted her examination. After noting the condition and treatment, she stored the computer file, looked at the list, got the next file.

When ten-year-old Damascus Geebel came in with a letter from her mother explaining that the girl had an ear infection, Neubach made a quick entry, looked in the girl's ear, prescribed an antibiotic (the prescription printed out automatically at the reception desk), and sent Damascus on her way.

Neubach dispatched flu, colds, sore throats, and the like in ten minutes or less. On average, patients waited about thirty minutes. No one seemed to mind the wait. Robert Grunen, a truck driver with back problems, said, "I've no reason to be dissatisfied. The care you get is very good." Gabriela Foitzik, a nursing home worker suffering from the flu, said, "My whole family goes to Dr. Neubach—husband, daughter, mother, sisters. . . . She's a good doctor."

Neither Grunen nor Foitzik has ever even seen a doctor's bill. The same holds true for most Germans. Doctors send their bills directly to the nonprofit sickness funds that insure virtually every German. These funds collect premiums through employer-employee contributions and then pay the doctors and hospitals. As far as the patient is concerned, it all happens automatically.

■

By the time Neubach drove off in her blue Volkswagen Rabbit to see the cancer patient, she had already treated thirty-one people for colds, flu, high blood pressure, pancreatitis, heart disease, and other complaints. The bedridden woman lived in a tiny apartment with her eleven-year-old son and seventy-four-year-old mother. "It is so sad," Neubach said.

Once inside the woman's bedroom, Neubach found herself faced with a problem—how to hang the bag for an intravenous solution. She hooked the plastic sack to a coat hanger and hung it from the ceiling light fixture. Neubach told her patient she would be back later that day and again the next. If she needed it, the doctor would give her an injection of morphine. "I want her to know that I'll be there for her," Neubach said. "We try to help the family keep someone terminally ill at home. It seems so much better to be with your loved ones than alone in a hospital room," she explained.

Such house calls aren't unique in Germany. Neubach makes visits between noon and three P.M. almost every day. "I like making house calls," she said. ". . . I get to meet the whole family, see the social situation. It is more personal."

Both Fleishman in the United States and Robinson in Canada make a limited number of house calls, primarily to elderly shut-ins. But Neubach makes all kinds of home visits. In fact, about once a month she is required by the regional physicians' association, as are all family practitioners, to serve a shift as a "taxi doctor." She rides around the whole Neuaubing area making house calls.

After leaving her cancer patient, Neubach had lunch in a local Italian restaurant, where she was warmly greeted by the owner, a patient, and then made two more house calls. She was back at her office by three P.M.

■

Again the waiting room was filled, mainly with minor complaints, because Germans, like Canadians, are quick to turn to the doctor. After all, it is free. On average, Germans go to the doctor about eleven times a year, almost twice as often as Americans.

"It seems that people in America are willing to take an active part in their health," said Neubach, who was born and raised in California before moving to Germany for medical school. "People here expect the medical system to fix things for them."

While Neubach dispatched the common cases quickly, her pace slowed when Maria Heller, seventy-five, came in to review some puzzling test results from a specialist. The diminutive woman had first come to Neubach after losing nearly twenty-six pounds over the previous year. The doctor's initial examination revealed nothing specific.

Neubach sent Heller to a pulmonologist for tests. They were inconclusive. Visits to a cardiologist and a neurologist

Comparing Doctor Care

Canada:
- All doctor visits free, including checkups.
- Number of doctor visits unlimited.
- Choice of doctors unlimited.
- Emphasis on primary care.

Germany:
- All doctor visits free, including checkups.
- Number of doctor visits unlimited.
- Choice of doctors unlimited.
- Family doctor referral needed to see specialists.
- House calls still common.

United States:
- Checkups not usually covered.
- Child immunizations often not covered.
- Routine doctor visits covered under HMOs.
- HMO and Medicaid patients limited in choice of doctors.
- Emphasis on specialized care.

followed. Their examinations were also inconclusive. At each step, however, it was Neubach who decided the next move and, in large part, what the specialists would do. "I can completely control it. That way I can work cost-effectively," she explained. "I can order a particular procedure from a specialist and no more, or simply refer her." This assures that blood work, X rays, and other tests won't be repeated by each specialist.

In Germany, a patient needs a referral from a family physician even to see a specialist. But Neubach said that she, like most primary-care doctors, never blocks a patient who insists on seeing a specialist. In Maria Heller's case, the weight loss remained a mystery, but no other adverse symptoms developed. "We will just have to keep an eye on it," Neubach said.

The elderly woman was satisfied. Dr. Neubach, she said, is a *"phantastischer Doktor."*

■

The German system requires Neubach to be a "gate-keeper" to the entire health-care apparatus and try to use its resources judiciously. In that effort, Neubach faces some built-in limitations and pressures.

Doctors' fees are negotiated between the insurance funds and the regional physicians' association, the Kassenärztliche Vereinigung. They agree on an annual lump-sum payment to the KV. This payment will cover all doctor visits for the year.

The KV disburses the money to doctors based on the number of examinations and procedures they do. (This fee-for-service approach is also how American and Canadian doctors charge.) If the volume of office visits, tests, and procedures jumps too much, the KV, which is dealing with a fixed pot of money, just cuts the size of each payment. A doctor who tries to boost income by ordering lots of tests and seeing lots of patients isn't milking "the system," but milking fellow doctors. Such behavior ultimately reduces every doctor's fees.

Therefore, it is the doctors' association, not the government, that rigorously monitors doctors' claims. Using a computerized system, the KV reviews each physician's practice from year to year and any drastic changes are quickly noted. "The KV monitors pharmaceutical use, hospital use, the number of cases," Neubach said, "and it can call an audit and go through all the cases at any time."

Neubach said that in 1991 she netted about $136,000 from her practice. She said her income has been growing because her practice has been growing.

Since there are a limited number of deutsche marks to be had, Neubach has an incentive to treat as many patients as she can and refer as few as possible to the specialists. She has a similar incentive to keep patients out of the hospital. German law prevents community-based doctors from practicing in hospitals, and hospital doctors (who are salaried) from working in the community. This is the great divide of German medical care.

"It is a shame," Neubach said. Often, tests are duplicated when a patient enters the hospital. And sometimes the hospitals "disregard the practitioner . . . and do something completely different," she said.

In response to the great divide, private practitioners offer a wide variety of services in oncology, radiology, and other medical specialties that, in the United States, are more generally found in hospitals. They also are willing to make more house calls and handle patients—such as someone dying of cancer—who would probably be hospitalized in the United States.

One other consequence of the great divide is that community doctors have virtually no allegiance to a particular hospital, the way doctors such as Fleishman do in the United States.

Germany's past efforts haven't been enough to hold down costs, so in 1992, an additional control was imposed on prescription drugs. Any physician prescribing more than $80,000 in pharmaceuticals had to pay the difference. This was done because Germans use so many prescription drugs—about twice as many, per capita, as Americans. So, doctors now have to balance the effectiveness of more expensive drugs against cheaper ones, and the needs of healthier patients against sicker ones.

But if a patient feels a doctor is being too stingy with drugs or services, he can freely switch physicians. And the competition among physicians is fierce. Medical education is free in Germany to every qualified student. This has led to an oversupply—there are about 30 percent more doctors per capita in Germany than in the United States.

■

By five P.M., Neubach had seen ten more patients, including seventeen-year-old Klute Arnberg. Several months earlier, Arnberg had broken his leg skiing in the Bavarian Alps. The fall also ruptured a benign cyst on his kidney. The cyst "swelled to the size of a cantaloupe. . . . It was a dangerous situation," Neubach said. It was successfully treated with antibiotics, and Neubach now does periodic ultrasound scans to check the cyst.

At six P.M., Neubach and Reidel reviewed the day's patients on the computer to make sure all the payment codings were correct. A total of seventy-six people had come in that day. Neubach had seen forty-two and also made three house calls.

On her way out, the phone rang. It was a patient with a case of arthritis so severe that Neubach had referred her to a rheumatologist. The woman was scheduled to enter the hospital the following day. But this evening the pain was too intense. Neubach told the woman's husband she would stop by on her way home—one more house call—and give the woman an injection of painkiller.

CHAPTER 3

BIRTH:
A DEFINING MOMENT
IN THE DELIVERY
OF HEALTH CARE

When Anne and Keith Bell arrived at Lankenau Hospital for the birth of their first baby, they headed off in opposite directions. Anne went to get admitted to maternity. Keith went to financial services, where he handed over a check for $225.

The Bells had been told that their insurance company would almost surely not cover their baby's birth. So for the previous seven months, the young couple had been diligently paying for the baby on the installment plan. The $225 was supposed to be their final payment. But a last-minute complication meant that the baby would be delivered by cesarean section—and that would add more to the bill.

Today, though, the Bells didn't have time to dwell on that. In a few hours, their baby would be born.

■

Of all the reasons for going to a hospital, none is so common as giving birth. Yet this universal life event is decidedly different depending on the country, and the health-care system, that you're in.

In America, the experience of giving birth is largely shaped by a woman's insurance status. If she is lucky enough, she'll have good insurance to pay the $4,500 average charge for prenatal care and birth. If she's poor enough, the government's Medicaid program will pick up the tab.

But for a growing number of American families who have no insurance or inadequate insurance, the joy of having a baby is tainted by financial worries. By one count, there are 14.6 million American women of childbearing age without insurance for maternity care. An American family can take home a baby and still be paying on the hospital bill when the child starts first grade.

That doesn't happen in Canada or Germany, where the government guarantees comprehensive medical care for everyone. If Anne Bell were a mother-to-be in Canada, her government health card would not only cover the delivery, it would get her all the prenatal care she needed, from the doctor of her choice. The same would be true in Germany. There, her doctor would even give her a blue booklet called a *Mutterpass*, to keep track of the many physical exams and medical tests offered to every pregnant woman.

If there is one area in which both nations far surpass the United States, it is in assuring that virtually every woman, rich or poor, gets the best possible chance for a healthy pregnancy. For its failure in this area, the United States pays a heavy price.

America's high-technology hospitals have become amazingly proficient at saving smaller and smaller babies. But the U.S. health-care system has made little progress in seeing that babies aren't born tiny and sickly in the first place. In fact, many American women face more hurdles than ever in getting good care during pregnancy.

This is a story of three women—Anne Bell, whose baby was born at Lankenau in suburban Philadelphia; Alice Chu, who gave birth at North York General Hospital in Toronto; and Silvana Dominelli, who had her baby at

Infant Mortality

Deaths in first year of life per 1,000 live births.

Canada	7.1
Germany	7.5
U.S.	8.9

SOURCE: UNICEF, 1991

Low Birthweight

Percent of infants born weighing less than 5 1/2 pounds.

Canada	6%
Germany	6%
U.S.	7%

SOURCE: UNICEF, 1991

Births in Three Countries

Canada:
- All prenatal care covered.
- All women free to choose doctor and hospital.
- All bills paid by government.
- Babies issued health card at birth.

Germany:
- All prenatal care covered.
- All women free to choose doctor and hospital.
- All bills paid by sickness funds; small co-payment for hospital.
- Most babies delivered by midwives.

United States:
- Coverage varies widely.
- Hundreds of thousands of women not covered at all.
- Many policies only partly cover prenatal care.
- Women with private insurance have wide choice of doctors.
- Poor women have fewer choices.

Schwabing Hospital in Munich. Their experiences in pregnancy and birth speak not just to the fundamental differences in the health-care systems of the United States, Canada, and Germany, but to the priorities that each country sets for the well-being of its families.

How a baby arrives in the world is only the beginning.

∎

 After Keith Bell returned from the business office, he and Anne, twenty-five, went up to maternity. She changed into a white hospital gown and coordinated robe printed with the Lankenau logo, and settled into her semi-private room. The Bells could hardly believe they had made it to this day, considering all that had come before.

Their problems began one day in January 1992 when they received a notice from Blue Cross/Blue Shield stating that their new policy would take effect February 1.

Keith, twenty-four, who works in the produce business, had recently switched jobs and health insurance policies. An insurance representative had told him in December that his new coverage would begin in January. Now, it turned out, he and Anne were looking at a one-month lapse in coverage.

A few days later, Anne took a home pregnancy test. It showed she was pregnant, a happy surprise. Then the couple remembered their insurance. "Oh, my God," Anne said, echoing what Keith was thinking. Could it be that she had gotten pregnant the one month they had no health insurance? In a panic, Anne phoned the office of Mark Chasteney, her doctor at Lankenau. Chasteney had delivered three of her sister's babies, and Anne had planned on having him deliver her children, too.

Anne explained her predicament to a billing clerk. The woman told Anne that her insurance would probably refuse to pay for the prenatal care and delivery on the grounds that her pregnancy was a "pre-existing condition." Many American insurance companies write this loophole into their policies for all sorts of problems. Without the insurance, the Bells would have to pay Chasteney's $2,200 obstetrics fee out of their own pockets. Of even greater concern was the hospital bill, which could easily total $5,000.

Anne burst into tears. There was no way she and her husband could afford that. She worked cutting hair and cleaning houses. She and Keith were living with his parents in Bryn Mawr while saving all they made to buy a house. Having a baby could leave them broke.

Chasteney's office suggested that Anne consider enrolling instead as a patient at the hospital's obstetrical clinic. The clinic would give her the same checkups and tests as a private doctor, but it would be cheaper. Staffed by young doctors in training, the clinic mostly serves poor women on Medicaid and those who have no health insurance. Lankenau has a policy of not turning any pregnant woman away.

Anne and Keith debated into the night whether to stay with Chasteney and take the gamble that Blue Cross/Blue Shield would in the end pay the bills, or play it safe and go to the clinic. "It was a nightmare for me," Anne would later say. "I was so glad we had found Mark Chasteney. He was so nice, so down to earth, so caring."

Still, they saw no choice: Anne enrolled in the clinic.

■

The morning light was just peeking through the windows of Schwabing Hospital in the heart of Munich when midwife Pia Diefenbacher took Silvana Dominelli under her wing.

Silvana, twenty-three, had arrived at Schwabing in the middle of the night, anxious and uncomfortable in the early stage of labor. This would be the second child for Silvana and her husband, Nazzareno, a construction worker, but they were no less excited than the first time.

They had chosen Schwabing, one of Munich's four city hospitals, because they had a good experience when their son, Carmello, was born here two years earlier. The hospital was old, and its maternity department lacked the niceties of some others—like the popular, ultramodern, high-tech Red Cross Hospital for Women. But Schwabing had an excellent reputation for infant care, and the Dominellis felt they'd be in good hands.

Costs never crossed their minds. The Dominellis were insured by Allgemeine Ortskrankenkasse (AOK), the largest of 1,200 "sickness funds" in Germany. Under the country's system of health care, virtually all Germans belong to a sickness fund, financed by joint contributions from workers and their employers. Employer and employee each contributes, on average, 6.25 percent of the worker's salary. AOK would cover all of Silvana's bills, except for an $8-a-day copayment on her hospital bill.

With her contractions growing stronger and more regular, Silvana was in a labor room on the third floor of Schwabing's Building VII, being coached reassuringly by midwife Diefenbacher. Unlike in the United States, where birth has become a big-ticket medical event directed by doctors and heavy on technology, birth in Germany is simple and natural. In Germany, under law, midwives deliver nearly all babies. Doctors get involved only in case of emergency.

From now until the baby was born, Diefenbacher would give Silvana her undivided attention. She had studied three years at the University of Freiburg to become a midwife and was committed to helping women get through labor with as little medical intervention as possible. "When I'm with a woman, I speak with her and I can look into her eyes," Diefenbacher said. "Then she does not so much need medication."

Diefenbacher sensed that Silvana was tense and tired and not so eager to cooperate. If only she could get her to relax, the labor would progress more smoothly. To help things along, the midwife suggested Silvana try a technique favored by German midwives: to sit with her legs spread on a huge, green plastic ball. Sitting on the ball would help relax the pelvic muscles and get the cervix to open.

Silvana's cervix was four centimeters dilated. That meant she still had six centimeters to go until she could begin to push. There was no telling how long that would take.

■

It was ten in the morning in Toronto, and thirty-year-old Alice Chu couldn't help but wonder whether her baby would ever be born. After a long and restless night and little progress in her labor, her husband, Gary, twenty-eight, had gone home for some sleep. Alice was momentarily alone with her pain.

She was in Labor Room 264 at North York General Hospital, a large community hospital on the northern outskirts of Toronto. Her room, on the second floor, was plain, with a bed, a vinyl-covered chair, a metal locker, and a sink. There was a TV and a bathroom across the hall.

Alice, who had come to the hospital nearly twenty hours before, was getting a drug called Pitocin to strengthen her contractions and help move her labor along. Because of the medication, she was hooked to an electronic fetal monitor to track contractions and the baby's heart rate. The monitor could be viewed remotely by nurses on duty at the desk in the hallway. The nurse assigned to Alice, Barb Stronach, periodically came into the room to look at the squiggly lines on the monitor's readout.

Alice had immigrated to Toronto from Hong Kong one-and-a-half years earlier to marry Gary, whom she had known since high school. An engineer for a telecommunications company, Gary had moved to Canada when he was sixteen.

Under Canadian law, Alice Chu—like all immigrants—was eligible to enroll in Ontario's health program within three months of establishing legal residency. Her red-and-white health card guaranteed that the government would cover virtually all her health-care costs, as it does for all Canadian citizens. She and Gary also had supplemental insurance provided by his company to pay for things they would not receive from the tax-financed, government-administered plan—prescription drugs, eyeglasses, and a semiprivate room instead of a standard four-person ward room.

When Alice became pregnant, the Chus' family doctor suggested she see a group practice of five obstetricians, whose offices were in a medical building adjacent to North York General. Although many Canadian GPs do obstetrics, Alice's did not. Alice chose the practice her doctor recommended because it included a woman doctor who spoke Chinese. It was a comfort knowing there was someone she could speak to in her native tongue should a concern arise.

She also was glad she picked North York because it was well known for its maternity care. It has one of the busiest wards in all of Canada, delivering about 3,600 babies a year. It also has a big genetics center for prenatal testing.

By 10:30, Alice's contractions were taking her breath away. The nurse asked if she wanted something for the pain. Alice said yes, and within minutes an anesthesiologist gave her an epidural anesthesia. It left her numb from the waist down.

Alice was smiling now, and Gary was back, his anxiety soothed by a bit of rest. "Can I have the baby soon?" she asked.

■

The World Health Organization says the well-being of a nation and the effectiveness of its health-care system can be measured, in part, by the health of the babies it brings into the world. By that measure, Canada and Germany are far better off than the United States.

When countries are ranked by the number of babies who survive their first year, Canada comes in ninth. Germany is fifteenth. The United States ranks twenty-third, according to 1991 data. The United States fares even worse in the number of low-birthweight babies. It ranks thirty-first.

Whether a baby is born healthy depends a lot on the quality of medical care the mother gets in pregnancy. In that regard, the United States again has a dismal record. Nearly one in three American women do not get adequate prenatal care, according to a report issued in February 1993 by the National Academy of Sciences' Institute of Medicine. Some pregnant women never see a doctor until they arrive at the hospital in labor.

Because so many American women don't get good prenatal care, more sickly, premature, and low-birthweight babies are born in the United States than in other industrialized nations. There are enormous social and economic costs.

These tiny babies are forty times more likely to die in the first four weeks of life. And even if medical technology saves them—at a cost of more than $1,000 a day in an intensive care nursery—they frequently face a lifetime of problems such as cerebral palsy, learning disabilities, and mental retardation. Hospital bills for these underweight babies total at least $2 billion a year.

The Institute of Medicine estimates that for every dollar society spends on prenatal care, it saves three dollars in medical costs later on, by detecting and managing problems that could lead to premature birth. Checkups—which include such simple things as weighing the pregnant woman, taking her blood pressure, measuring her abdomen, and testing her urine—can make an enormous difference. They can pinpoint a baby's failure to grow, as well as pregnancy-induced diabetes or other conditions that lead to premature birth. Good nutrition, vitamins, and counseling on the dangers of drinking, smoking, and drug abuse can help prevent underweight babies, respiratory and developmental problems in babies, and fetal alcohol syndrome. Screening the mother for syphilis can prevent birth defects. Genetic testing can detect inherited diseases.

Despite overwhelming evidence that prenatal care makes a big difference, the United States has no public policy to ensure that all pregnant women get it. To the contrary, financial barriers often work against a woman's best intentions. This is especially so for the 555,000 women who give birth each year without insurance. These women account for about one in every seven births. Private physicians often won't take them as patients unless they pay hundreds of dollars up front.

A study in March 1993 in the *Journal of the American Medical Association* reported that women with no health coverage were two-and-a-half times more likely than privately insured women to postpone care until the end of pregnancy. They were six times more likely to get no care at all. Even women whose maternity costs are paid by Medicaid may have trouble finding a doctor, because obstetricians complain they don't get reimbursed enough to take these women as patients.

Such problems do not exist in Canada and Germany. Universal health coverage and standard reimbursement rates for doctors make it rare that a pregnant woman goes without regular checkups.

In Germany, "there is simply never a question of whether a pregnant woman has easy access to the care she needs, and there is never a question of proof of payment for those services," said Dr. C. Arden Miller, a pediatrician and professor at the University of North Carolina, Chapel Hill, who has studied maternity care in ten European countries.

His study of Germany found that 98 percent of pregnant women arrive at the hospital with their *Mutterpass* at the time of delivery. The thirty-two-page booklet, designed by physicians and insurance funds in 1985, becomes a record for all the exams and tests a woman gets, including at least ten prenatal visits, two ultrasound scans, and any necessary lab work.

In Canada, even immigrant women, often poor and coping with language difficulties, rarely miss prenatal care. Dr. Dennis Xuereb, the North York obstetrician who would deliver Alice Chu's baby, said his waiting room was evidence of the single standard of care that exists for every woman—regardless of income or status.

"We have Somalian refugees. We have Sri Lankan refugees. We have Chinese refugees. We have lawyers, engineers, we have every cross-section you can imagine," Xuereb said. "Every single patient is treated the same way and has the right to the same care."

■

By the time Anne Bell was admitted to Lankenau's maternity ward, she and Keith had paid well over $1,000. When Anne enrolled as a clinic patient, the couple had to sign a contract with the hospital promising to pay $975 in advance of the birth. On top of that, the Bells had paid $185 for various medical tests, and they owed hundreds more for other lab bills and procedures.

In the meantime, they were continuing to pay $293 a month on their Blue Cross/Blue Shield policy. Keith was holding out hope that their insurance would come through for them after the baby was born, but many calls to Blue Cross and Blue Shield had yielded conflicting and confusing information.

At his old job, Keith could turn to a company worker who handled insurance matters. But now that he and Anne were insured under an individual policy, they were on their own. The complexities of health insurance, Keith had discovered, were mind-boggling.

While Keith worried about finances, Anne had immersed herself in preparing for childbirth. Her last prenatal visit to the hospital's obstetrical clinic had been five days before she delivered.

Clinic B at Lankenau Hospital didn't open for business until nine A.M. that day. But more than an hour before, Anne, dressed in a gray velour sweatsuit, lowered herself into one of the dozens of chairs lined up in the empty waiting room. By then, Anne knew the clinic routine well.

Waiting was part of the game. She had learned to get there early and sign in, so she would be the first in and the first out.

Anne was anxious for one last talk with Douglas Coslett, the doctor who would be doing the delivery. Coslett, in his last year of training in obstetrics, had gotten to know Anne and her insurance predicament. She was happy to have finally developed rapport with a particular doctor because she had felt embarrassed by the clinic routine of being examined by a different person nearly every time she came in.

It was Coslett who had told her the baby would be born by cesarean section because it was in the breech position, feet-first instead of head-down. Doctors are reluctant to deliver such a baby vaginally, especially a first baby, because they fear complications.

While Anne waited for the clinic to open, she remembered she had some financial matters to deal with. She went upstairs to meet with Patti Yost, in the hospital's financial services department. It was Yost's job to deal with patients coming into the hospital with no insurance or inadequate coverage.

She pulled the Bells' file and looked it over. Now that Anne needed a C-section, another $225 would be added to the bill, Yost explained.

"This has to be paid before you deliver," Yost said.

Anne was taken aback. "I didn't realize this was all due before I deliver."

Yost reminded her that she was getting a bargain. Her birth, she said, would actually cost about $8,000. Then, Yost reconsidered. Because Anne had just learned she needed a C-section, Yost gave her thirty days after the birth to pay the extra money. She handed Anne a pre-addressed envelope for mailing the payment.

Anne returned to the clinic to wait. Shortly before nine, a nurse called her into an examining room, weighed her, and checked her blood pressure.

Anne's medical chart served as another reminder of her standing in the eyes of the health-care system. It bore the words: "Self Pay."

■

Once the time comes to deliver, Lankenau offers every expectant mother the same high-quality, high-technology care. It doesn't matter what her insurance status is.

In each of the hospital's six labor-delivery-recovery rooms, there are fetal monitors, automatic pumps for epidurals and intravenous lines, machinery to measure blood pressure and pulse, and newborn warming beds equipped for any emergency.

The technology is complemented by such amenities as showers, TVs with a special channel on parenting issues, and easy chairs for expectant dads. A soft color theme of peaches and greens is repeated in the wallpaper, carpets, and accessories in patient rooms and delivery areas.

There are other touches. Lankenau sends new parents home with a thirty-dollar gift certificate to an area restaurant. It used to treat new parents to a surf-and-turf dinner in the hospital. But in 1992, Lankenau decided that, with insurance companies pressuring hospitals to shorten a new mother's stay, patients weren't around long enough to enjoy a celebratory dinner.

Having a first-rate delivery suite is a source of pride to Lankenau's medical and nursing staff, and it is critical to Lankenau's ability to stay competitive in a region packed with top-notch hospitals. But all the technology and extras come at a cost. According to Independence Blue Cross, Lankenau's average charge for a vaginal delivery in 1991— not including doctors' fees—was $6,153.

At North York General in Toronto, frills simply don't exist. The blueprints for a new maternity ward have been hanging on the wall of the doctors' lounge for so long that the paper is yellowing. The plans call for construction of modern labor-delivery-recovery rooms. Right now, women labor in one room and are wheeled across the hall into an old-fashioned delivery room to have the baby.

"We've been talking about it for ten years," said Xuereb, Alice Chu's doctor. Renovations were scheduled to begin in the fall of 1993.

For each delivery, the hospital spends $800 of its annual budget, which was $79 million in 1992. That unyielding annual budget, set by the provincial government, forces the administration to make hard choices. In one recent money-saving move, North York began asking new mothers to bring a supply of diapers and sanitary napkins when they come in to have their babies.

The hospital management sees that as a small trade-off for keeping its commitment to quality medical care. For instance, North York is so committed to the benefits of breast-feeding that it refuses gift packs from formula companies and routinely keeps a woman in the hospital longer if she's having trouble breast-feeding. A public-health nurse also visits new mothers at home, if needed.

At Schwabing, in Munich, the reliance on midwives and women's preference for natural childbirth help limit the cost. The hospital has available the same technology found in Canada and the United States, but it isn't used nearly as extensively.

Just 8 percent of women who deliver at Schwabing request an epidural to deaden pain. At North York, 60 percent of women get this expensive procedure, requiring an anesthesiologist. At Lankenau, 80 percent get it, adding about $600 to the bill.

After the birth, German women are given much more time to recuperate. New mothers typically stay in the hospital six days, a recuperation the Germans call *Wochenbett,* or "week in bed." The sickness fund picks up the cost at a flat rate of $344 a day at Schwabing. Canadian and American mothers are typically on their way home after two nights.

■

By 9:30 A.M., Silvana Dominelli's labor had progressed to the point that she had been moved from a labor room at Schwabing to an old-fashioned operating-delivery room. It was massive, with just a delivery table at the far end near the windows. A white screen shielded the view from the door.

Silvana was hooked up to a monitor to track contractions and fetal heart rate. The thump-thump-thump of the monitor echoed through the big room. With the midwife's help, Silvana still was going without painkilling drugs, despite strong contractions caused by Pitocin, the labor-inducing drug she was getting.

Midwife Diefenbacher would be backed up by Dr. Gilbert Schmid, a tall, thin man who is assistant to the chief of obstetrics at Schwabing. Silvana had brought her *Mutterpass,* a helpful reference for Diefenbacher and Schmid, who had never seen Silvana before. The German system of medicine draws a sharp division between doctors who work in the community and those who work in the hospital. The doctor who gave Silvana eight months of prenatal care would not deliver her baby.

"Now it is time to start pushing," Diefenbacher told Silvana, who clung to her husband for support. "Breathe . . . breathe . . . close your mouth . . . push . . . push."

Silvana was doing the pushing, but Diefenbacher was working hard, too. Her face dripped with sweat. Wisps of hair fell around her face as she coached Silvana.

Schmid was also encouraging Silvana to push. He commended her husband, Nazzareno, for being a good helper. Nazzareno bent close each time his wife had a contraction and allowed her to cling desperately to his neck.

Schmid periodically checked the printout on the fetal monitor. After one check, he talked quietly with Diefenbacher. Silvana had been pushing for twenty minutes with little progress. There were signs that the baby's heart rate was slowing. They decided to speed up the delivery by using a technique called vacuum extraction.

A second midwife was called in. Diefenbacher told Silvana to push as the second midwife pressed on her belly. When the head was visible in the birth canal, Schmid placed the suction cup on it and, using vacuum pressure, gently eased the baby out.

At one minute of ten, Diefenbacher held up Baby Girl Dominelli. Silvana could barely draw the strength to look, but Nazzareno beamed at his new daughter. Diefenbacher carried her to a counter, cleaned her up, weighed her, and put a pink bracelet on her left wrist.

Schmid looked over the baby. He agreed with the midwife's assessment that the baby was too pale. Diefenbacher threaded a tiny tube down the baby's windpipe and then sucked on the other end to clear mucus out of the airways. Soon, a pediatrician arrived to have a look.

■

Alice Chu was exhausted. She had labored twenty-four hours at the Toronto hospital. Finally, she was ready to push. She was rolled into the delivery room at 2:45 P.M., as her husband, Gary, hurriedly covered his clothes with a green surgical gown. Working the delivery would be two nurses, an anesthesiologist, and Xuereb, the obstetrician.

Between the numbing effects of the epidural and her fatigue, Alice was having trouble pushing. Xuereb was not particularly worried. He had decided to use forceps to help things along. "You all right, Mrs. Chu?" he asked. "You'll feel a little bit of pain. You'll know I'm doing something, but it won't hurt. We're going to ask you to push and help us."

On each contraction, Xuereb told Chu to push. He and nurse Stronach encouraged her to stick with it. "It takes more than one push," he said. "You're fine. We'll take our time doing it."

He picked up the metal forceps, which looked like hinged salad tongs, slid them around the baby's head, and gently guided the baby out.

"Almost there . . . last effort . . . there we go. . . . Are you ready for motherhood?"

"It's a girl," he said, holding up a baby with thick, dark hair.

Gary looked at his daughter and asked, "Is she normal?"

■

A cloud hangs over every birth: the parents' fear that their child will be less than perfect. In the United States, there's another cloud: the doctor's fear that—whether he was at fault or not—he will be sued.

In Canada or Germany, a somewhat difficult birth might be helped along with techniques such as forceps. In the United States, such a birth is apt to become a major surgical event. Nearly one in every four babies in the United States is delivered by cesarean section. In Canada, the rate is one in five babies. In Germany, only one in seven babies is born surgically.

The volume of C-sections in the United States has been the single most debated issue surrounding childbirth since the early 1970s. Although it spares the baby a possibly traumatic birth, it is riskier for the mother. The procedure involves a major cut to the abdomen, with risk of infection and bleeding. And it lays the mother up for weeks afterward, often interfering with her ability to care for her newborn.

The widespread practice of C-sections is also controversial because of the cost. In 1991, the average hospital charge for a normal delivery in Philadelphia was $4,579. For a C-section, it was $9,359.

All those C-sections add up. A study released in April

1993 by the federal Centers for Disease Control and Prevention found that, nationwide, doctors performed 349,000 unnecessary C-sections in 1991, at an added cost of about $1 billion in doctor and hospital charges. The report noted that the operation is performed more often on well-insured women.

"When the malpractice issue became a huge one, we began to do things in the hope of preventing a malpractice action against us. Those things became habit," said Dr. Kaighn Smith, head of obstetrics and gynecology at Lankenau Hospital. "The C-section became standard of care."

Eighty percent of U.S. obstetricians have been sued at least once, according to a survey by the American College of Obstetricians and Gynecologists. Awards to parents can go into the millions.

Doctors can be sued in Germany and Canada, but lawsuits are not as common, the awards tend not to be as high, and insurance premiums are lower. An obstetrician in Canada pays about $14,000 for malpractice insurance, compared with $37,000 in the United States.

Malpractice premiums, according to the Congressional Budget Office, total less than 1 percent of the U.S. health bill. Some contend there is a ripple effect that is far costlier because doctors practice "defensive medicine." Not taking a chance may mean ordering more lab tests and X rays or more consultations with specialists.

In obstetrics, this type of medicine can lead to a greater reliance on fetal monitoring, even though there is no evidence to prove that routine monitoring improves the chances of a healthy birth. It can mean turning more quickly to a C-section, rather than using mechanical aids such as forceps, if labor is not progressing or the fetal monitor suggests some irregularity in the baby's heartbeat.

Roger Freeman, a California obstetrician who headed a national committee to set standards for the use of forceps, said that forceps unfairly got a bad name years ago after research reported that their use could cause physical and mental defects. "I did a forceps delivery not long ago and the nurse turned to me and said, 'I didn't think we did those anymore,'" said Freeman. More recent studies disprove the earlier findings and indicate that forceps are safe in the hands of doctors trained to use them.

Dr. Mel Petersiel, chief of obstetrics at North York General, said forceps are involved in 20 percent of North York's deliveries. Their use helps keep the hospital's C-section rate to about 16 percent, lower even than the national average.

At Lankenau, where 5 percent of births in 1992 were by forceps, 25 percent of babies were delivered by C-section.

■

It was 12:20 P.M. when Anne Bell was wheeled into Lankenau's operating room No. 1. She giggled nervously as she sat on the edge of the operating table, waiting for the anesthesiologist.

The room was awash in bright light and filled with equipment. The birth would be staffed by eight people: four nurses; Dr. Coslett, who would be doing the delivery; another resident, Dr. Virginia Ferlan; Dr. John DeMaio, the hospital's chief of neonatology; and Dr. John Sauter, the anesthesiologist.

As the nurses laid out the surgical tools, Coslett came breezing in, quipping, "Anyone here with an upside-down baby, ready to have one?" Before the operation began, the doctors used ultrasound to take one last look at whether the baby had flipped into a head-first position. The baby hadn't.

From there, things moved swiftly. At 1:27, with Anne anesthetized from the waist down and Keith sitting nervously near her head, the operation began. Coslett made an incision in her abdomen.

It was 1:33 on the operating room clock when Baby Bell

was born. "Have a look," said Coslett, lifting the eight-pound, two-ounce baby. "It's a boy."

The Bells named him James Martin. That was in honor of Anne's father, and her brother, who died when he was eight.

■

The Chus' baby girl wasn't an hour old when she was issued her very own health card, taped to her bassinet. Baby Chu was now not only a citizen of Canada but also a brand-new member of the nation's health-care system. The temporary card—to be replaced by a permanent one within six weeks—would allow her parents to take her to a doctor of their choice for checkups and shots. There would never be a question as to whether her parents could afford that care.

"If you look at all the systems in the world that address the needs of children, this is one of the best," said Jonathan Tolkin, chief of pediatrics at North York. "If you're a child coming into the world, you're given the best chance possible."

Under Canadian law, new mothers who work can take up to twenty-five weeks of paid leave at 57 percent of their weekly salary.

Alice Chu stayed in the hospital two nights. The baby checked out perfectly. She and Gary gave her the English name Jennifer and the Chinese name Lap-Man. They decided she had Gary's mouth, but her nose and eyes were Alice's.

■

Silvana Dominelli spent her six-day *Wochenbett* in the hospital. During that time, she had the option of attending exercise classes each day in the hospital's gymnasium. Mothers are encouraged to begin working out twenty-four hours after giving birth.

The Dominellis named their baby Giuseppina. Because

of the baby's paleness, doctors initially worried that she might have an infection, but that didn't turn out to be the case.

The Dominellis took their daughter home to their small apartment in a neighborhood near the hospital. If they developed concerns about their baby, a public health nurse would come to their home. They left the hospital with a yellow booklet called a *Kinderpass* that would keep track of their daughter's childhood exams and vaccines just as Silvana's *Mutterpass* documented her pregnancy.

In Germany and Canada, about 85 percent to 90 percent of children are up to date on their shots. In the United States, the federal CDC says that only about half of two-year-olds are fully vaccinated. Because insurance policies often do not pay for vaccines and many young families do not have insurance anyway, President Clinton, early in his administration, proposed a program to provide free shots to all children.

Silvana was a homemaker. Had she been a working mother, she would have gotten a six-week paid leave before the birth and eight weeks afterward. Then, she could have taken three years off work, without pay, and be guaranteed her job back. This period of leave for new mothers to nurture their children is called an "education holiday."

The German government gives families monthly stipends of up to $372 per child, depending on their income, for at least one-and-a-half years to help in the raising of their children.

Nazzareno Dominelli said the birth couldn't have gone more smoothly. And he was happy to now have a daughter as well as a son. "I think this is just about perfect," he said.

■

Three days after the birth of baby James, Anne Bell got a message to call Patti Yost in the financial services office. Yost wanted to update Anne on the status of her insurance coverage. As she had explained before, she told Anne that it was unlikely Blue Cross would cover the bill. Even if the insurance company did eventually pay, it would probably take months to recoup the money.

Anne listened and hung up the phone. She was feeling tired, sore from her surgery, and anxious about her new role of mother. Somehow, she figured, she and Keith would pay their bills.

■

In January 1993, after Keith had called Blue Cross more than a dozen times, the Bells got word that it would cover Anne's hospital bill after all. Lankenau refunded to the Bells $475 of the money they had paid up front.

By April, seven months after James's birth, the Bells were still waiting to hear whether Blue Shield would pay the $667 in laboratory and medical testing bills from Anne's pregnancy.

CHAPTER 4
TECHNOLOGY: THE BOON AND BANE OF MEDICINE

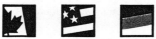

The X rays of Anthony Cavallaro's cardiovascular system looked terrible. All the major vessels that fed blood to his heart were clogged. The seventy-one-year-old man probably would not live long if something wasn't done to restore the flow. "You've got to do what you've got to do," the retired truck driver told doctors at Lankenau Hospital when they explained the gravity of his situation. Heart surgery was quickly scheduled. It would be done in two days.

Cavallaro could get this kind of care—the moment he needed or wanted it—because he lives in the United States. Almost all other nations try to curb the use of expensive, high-tech procedures such as heart surgery, to keep down medical costs. Canada and Germany long ago decided that hard choices had to be made, and limits had to be set on technology, even if it sometimes forced patients to wait for elective surgery, MRI (magnetic resonance imaging) exams, or heart stress tests.

Not so in the United States. Driven by the competitive forces of one of the few remaining free-market medical

Technology in Three Countries

Canada:
- Long waiting lists for some high-tech procedures.
- Government limits proliferation of technology.
- Patients sometimes must travel to get high-tech care.

Germany:
- Patients have less access to high-tech procedures.
- Government limits proliferation of technology.
- Patients sometimes must travel to get high-tech care.

United States:
- High-tech procedures readily available.
- No limits on spread of technology.

systems, U.S. medical centers have amassed an awesome collection of costly medical devices and specialists trained to use them. Philadelphia, one of the world's top medical centers, has almost an embarrassment of riches—so plentiful that roadside billboards advertise the high-tech wonders available in even the smallest hospitals.

In 1993, Philadelphia hospitals had sixty-three MRIs—compared with fifty-seven in all of Germany and just twelve in all of Canada. Philadelphia-area hospitals had seventy-one CAT scan machines, fifteen nurseries capable of caring for the tiniest of babies, and twenty-two organ-transplant programs. And Philadelphia had five times as many open-heart surgery programs as comparable cities in Canada or Germany.

This massive array, poised waiting to be used, is expensive in its own right—an MRI machine can cost up to $3 million. Once it's in use, even more costs are generated, because doctors tend to order more tests and other procedures, requiring more nurses and technicians, before they make a diagnosis or complete a treatment.

The Congressional Budget Office estimates that technology, and the increase it fosters in the intensity of care, is a major reason medical costs are rising so much faster than other segments of the U.S. economy. Yet there is no evidence that, for all this spending, Americans are doing any better medically.

■

Cavallaro, already heavily sedated, was taken on a litter to the Lankenau Hospital operating room at 7:45 A.M. It was a large, square, brightly lit room. Cavallaro was transferred to the operating table, surrounded by surgical equipment and electronic monitoring devices stacked so high that they towered above some of the shorter members of the surgical team.

There were a defibrillator to restart Cavallaro's heart with a jolt of electricity, a balloon pump to help it pump blood, an electrical cauterizing device to stop small, severed blood vessels from bleeding, and two computerized pumps to administer drugs in precise amounts. At the head of the table, the anesthetist station looked like the cockpit of a 747, with video tubes and dials and devices that would run four different drugs into Cavallaro's system to keep him in a deep sleep for the five-hour operation. To the side of the operating table was a low-lying machine with dials and whirring wheels. This was the heart-lung machine, the breakthrough technological advance that made heart surgery like this possible.

By 8:20, everything was ready for the senior surgeon, Scott M. Goldman. A nurse went over to Cavallaro, who was very drowsy. "We're going to call Dr. Goldman now, and then we're going to put you to sleep," she said. Cavallaro nodded.

Cavallaro's heart had been seriously damaged by a heart attack eighteen years earlier. Further weakened by atherosclerosis, a buildup of plaque in the blood vessels, it was pumping 50 percent less blood than normal. Without surgery, Goldman said, Cavallaro had a 20 percent chance of living five more years.

With Bruce Springsteen playing on a portable CD, Goldman made the first chest incision at 9:20. It took him an hour and twenty minutes to cut through tissue and muscle, open the rib cage, and reach the beating heart, moist and glistening under the overhead lights.

At 10:42, Goldman called for the heart-lung machine. Cavallaro's blood was immediately diverted through plastic tubes to the device, which oxygenated the blood and pumped it back into his body. Cavallaro's heart was stopped with the injection of a drug. Using sections of vein taken from Cavallaro's leg and a mammary artery from inside Cavallaro's chest, Goldman constructed new routes for the blood to take around the obstructions in the three coronary arteries.

At 11:54, the heart-lung machine was shut off, and the blood was rerouted through Cavallaro's heart, which started beating on its own. Twenty-five minutes later, Goldman was outside in the waiting area talking to Cavallaro's wife, Mary, and his daughter, Rosemarie McCloy.

"Everything went very nicely," Goldman said as the women looked up at him with concern from their seats in the hallway. "He had no trouble coming off of the machine. He's all right. He's fine."

With tears streaming down her face, Mary Cavallaro stood and hugged Goldman, who tensed from the sudden display of emotion.

"God bless you," McCloy said.

"I think he's going to do fine," Goldman said.

■

Heart bypass surgery could stand as a metaphor for what's good and what's bad about American medicine: It shows the immense power of medical technology—a technology that lets doctors shut off hearts and turn them back on, a technology that restores people crippled by heart disease to an active life. But it costs a fortune. In 1992, the

United States spent more than $6 billion—0.8 percent of its entire medical bill—on this one procedure, an operation that wasn't even possible a generation ago.

Since it was first done successfully at the Cleveland Clinic in 1967, heart bypass has become one of the nation's most common surgical procedures. More than 265,000 Americans had bypasses in 1991, at a cost of about $25,000 each. Canada doesn't do nearly as many. Bernard S. Goldman, head of cardiovascular surgery at Sunnybrook Health Science Centre in Toronto, said Canada performs sixty-five heart bypass operations per 100,000 population, while the United States does 125. Germany does forty-eight bypasses per 100,000.

U.S. doctors are much more aggressive in searching for clogged arteries and encouraging patients to undergo surgery, Goldman said, while Canadian doctors are more inclined to treat the problem with drugs and lifestyle changes such as exercise, cessation of smoking, or retirement.

The victims of heart attacks—or people suspected of having a heart attack—get particularly aggressive treatment in the United States. The U.S. doctor is more likely to admit patients with chest pain to the intensive care unit, more likely to prescribe drugs, and more likely to order X-ray angiography to look inside coronary arteries, according to a study cowritten by Jean L. Rouleau of the University of Sherbrooke, Quebec. The study, reported in March 1993 in the *New England Journal of Medicine,* also found that U.S. heart-attack victims are almost three times more likely than Canadians to go on to bypass surgery.

Does this mean Americans are getting too many operations, or Canadians are getting too few? No one knows. Despite the extra care American heart patients receive, Rouleau's study concluded that they did no better than Canadian patients. They were no more likely to avoid a second heart attack or to live longer. The only disadvantage of their conservative treatment was that Canadians were slightly more likely to experience the chest pain *angina pectoris.*

Goldman said the Canadian heart patients who don't get bypass surgery still enjoy a high quality of life, though they must take drugs or limit their activity more than those who have had the surgery. He scoffed at reports in the United States that some Canadians live painful, debilitated lives—or even die—while waiting for surgery. He said Canadian doctors are less likely than their American counterparts to encourage surgery for elderly patients with other incapacitating diseases such as arthritis.

"You've had an explosion of technology [in the United States] that has to be used and paid for," Goldman said. "And you have a completely entrepreneurial practice mode that is also sharply driven by litigation, that pushes the system. . . . People demand care, and doctors and hospitals are delighted to give care."

Scott Goldman, Cavallaro's surgeon and chief of the division of thoracic and cardiovascular surgery at Lankenau, agreed that American patients are more likely to demand surgery than Canadians. "I spend more time talking people out of surgery than urging patients to get it," he said. "People don't want to put up with symptoms in this country. . . . They are more likely to want an operation, and they want it yesterday."

■

In July 1992, heart-attack patient William E. Sequin, who lives in the small Canadian resort town of Orillia, about one hundred miles north of Toronto, underwent X-ray angiography to see if his coronary arteries were blocked. The sixty-five-year-old factory worker didn't have to worry about the cost of his care because Canada's national health insurance, funded from taxes, pays all doctor and hospital bills.

Sequin was becoming increasingly incapacitated by heart

disease. He no longer could walk more than a block or two without stopping or taking nitroglycerin pills to open his blood vessels and temporarily restore blood flow to his heart. The X-ray angiography showed that all three of Sequin's coronary arteries were blocked. Not enough blood was getting through to nourish his heart.

Eight days later, Sequin was sitting in the elegantly appointed offices of the chief of cardiac surgery at Sunnybrook, one of Canada's largest medical teaching institutions. Bernard S. Goldman told Sequin he needed bypass surgery but that his condition was neither an emergency nor urgent. He was not in imminent danger of a heart attack. He was classified as an "elective priority."

Elective-priority patients are supposed to be operated on within six weeks, Goldman said, but Sequin put the surgery off for personal reasons, and then Goldman went on vacation. In the United States, Sequin probably would have been operated on within a couple of weeks, if not immediately.

It wasn't until September 28, almost three months after his talk with Goldman, that Sequin received a letter from Sunnybrook saying that he had been scheduled for surgery.

Sequin arrived at Sunnybrook on October 14, eight days before surgery, for the patient orientation program, similar to those provided by many hospitals in the United States, including Lankenau. Seventeen men and women, most of them patients, were seated at three long tables. They ranged in age from thirty-two to seventy-two.

"We know there's a lot of anxiety about the surgery," said clinical nurse specialist Darlene Rebeyka, after welcoming the people to Sunnybrook. "It's the fear of the unknown. Sometimes people have a lot of unrealistic information from friends."

She gave everyone a booklet put out by the hospital. She played a videotape, which showed energetic people doing calisthenics, swimming, playing golf, and having a grand time after bypass surgery. The authoritative and friendly face of Bernard Goldman came on the screen. He talked about the technical aspects of heart surgery, and someone else provided reassuring statistics. Ninety-eight percent of patients survive surgery. Chest pain and all other symptoms are eliminated in 90 percent of patients. Two-thirds of patients no longer need heart drugs.

As the tape ended, eight women entered the room and identified themselves as part of the team that would care for the patients when they returned for surgery. There was an ICU nurse, floor nurse, nutritionist, pharmacist, occupational therapist, social worker, research nurse, and someone to coordinate the services.

After the presentation, a few questions were asked, the patients were urged to call if they had concerns, and then everyone left. Sequin drove home, greatly reassured. As far as he was concerned, the medical care system in Canada was just fine.

■

The waiting list that Sequin was on is part of Ontario's cardiac-care network. It was started in April 1991, after widely publicized reports that a handful of patients had died while waiting for heart surgery. The government also authorized an additional bypass program in Toronto, the one Goldman now heads at Sunnybrook. The government agreed to pay Sunnybrook for 635 procedures a year, increasing the number of heart operations in Toronto by 20 percent.

The cardiac waiting list ranks patients in four categories: Emergency (surgery should be done within twenty-four hours), Urgent (within fourteen days), Elective Priority (within six weeks), and Elective (within three months). Patients are periodically checked to make sure their conditions remain stable. Those who have deteriorated are moved to the top of the list. Because Sunnybrook is highly regarded for its heart surgery, and attracts a lot of patients, its three-month waiting period is longer than Ontario's average of about nine weeks.

Few patients needing heart surgery are so sick that they must have it immediately. "Hysteria is built into the U.S. system, with patients being rushed into surgery," Sunnybrook's Goldman said.

Despite the expanded heart program in Ontario, five Sunnybrook heart patients have died while waiting during a recent eighteen-month period. In that time, eight hundred patients got surgery.

How would Anthony Cavallaro have fared in Canada? He would have been classified as an urgent patient, just as he was at Lankenau, and operated on within fourteen days, according to waiting-list protocol, Bernard Goldman said. In Philadelphia, Cavallaro waited only two days.

■

William Sequin was relaxed on the morning of his surgery, having just gotten a shot of morphine and another drug. He was lying in bed, arms folded behind his head, joking with his five grown sons and daughters.

Two of Sequin's sons had driven him to the hospital the day before, making the hundred-mile trip in a little over two hours. Sequin had decided to go to a Toronto heart hospital because it was the closest to his home. He was free to pick any hospital he wanted, but only three hospitals in Toronto could offer him bypass surgery.

Germans are similarly free to pick hospitals, but they also have limited choices. Munich has only three adult heart programs. In the United States, hospitals doing bypass surgery are much more plentiful. When Cavallaro picked Lankenau, he chose from a list of sixteen adult heart programs in the Philadelphia area.

The litter for Sequin arrived at 1:10 P.M. After he kissed each of his children, Sequin was taken to a large operating room on the seventh floor with big picture windows. The equipment—monitoring devices and cathode tubes stacked one on top of the other, drug pumps, and the low-lying heart-lung machine to the side of the operating table—looked just like the setup in Lankenau.

The operation took a little more than four hours. When it ended, Sequin was taken to an eight-bed coronary-care unit and put in a corner bed, next to a picture window with a view of the city's skyscrapers in the distance.

■

Sequin's experience was not unlike that of retired Munich tailor Jakob Dobler, sixty-eight, who had come to Grosshadern Clinic at the University of Munich for a bypass operation. Dobler also had to wait months for his surgery because he was not considered sick enough for a high-priority classification. Just as at Sunnybrook, three months is the average wait at Grosshadern for elective heart surgery, said Bruno Reichart, the hospital's chief of heart surgery.

Dobler, a short, balding man with eyeglasses and a shy smile, said he had not had serious symptoms while waiting for his surgery. But now that it was about to happen, he was anxious to get it over with.

Dobler was sitting up in bed in a narrow room in the university hospital. The room was simple and clean, with a telephone and a connecting bathroom but no decorating flourishes. Two other patients shared his room.

Dobler had entered the hospital eight days earlier to start preoperative tests. He'd taken many of the tests before, but Reichart wanted to repeat them. So many weeks can pass between a patient's diagnosis and surgery that surgeons want to make sure nothing has changed.

Dobler belongs to one of Germany's 1,200 nonprofit "sickness funds," which cover 90 percent of Germans and pay for comprehensive in-hospital and outpatient medical care. The sickness funds are supported by contributions averaging 12.5 percent of a worker's salary, with the employer paying half this bill. The government pays the premiums for the unemployed.

A few floors below Dobler, Manfred Eisenbach also waited for heart surgery. Forty-eight years old and the owner of a roofing company in Plettenberg, a small community four hundred miles northwest of Munich, Eisenbach is one of the 10 percent of Germans who opt out of the sickness funds to buy private insurance.

Private insurance in Germany makes less difference in the care patients get than it does in the United States. Privately insured Americans have many more options than low-income people on Medicaid or those with no insurance at all, who are severely limited in their choices.

In Germany, sickness-fund patients can choose any primary physician they want and go to any hospital, just like the privately insured patients can. The advantage that privately insured patients have is that they get slightly more comfortable private or semiprivate rooms and can choose to be treated by the chief of the department. Private patients also get somewhat faster service. In Munich, their average wait for elective heart surgery is one month, instead of three. If the need for surgery is urgent, however, private and sickness-fund patients have equally fast access to care, Reichart said. As it turned out, Dobler and Eisenbach both ended up with the same surgeon—Reichart, the chief of surgery.

Dobler's five-hour operation went without incident. After surgery he was taken to the intensive care unit. The next day he was transferred to a nearby hospital to recover; his bed in Grosshadern Clinic was taken by a seventeen-year-old heart-transplant patient.

Although practically unheard of in the United States, the inter-hospital transfer of patients just before or after major surgery is not uncommon in Germany. There is such a demand for surgery at Munich's three heart centers that surgeons will operate even if they have to send patients to another hospital to recover. Sometimes surgeons will transfer patients who are still on ventilators.

Reichart said everyone who needs heart surgery gets it, though perhaps not as fast as they'd like. Rather than wait, many patients will fly to Switzerland or other countries that can offer heart surgery with less delay. The bills are paid by the German sickness funds.

Backlogs for heart surgery will be significantly relieved, Reichart said, when his program doubles in size in 1994. Until then, his team is doing 2,000 heart operations a year, including transplants. He said it took him a year to persuade government and university officials to spend $16.8 million on expansion. Reichart argued for more capacity so he could reduce the waiting time to one month, and also so he could serve many of the patients who go out of the country for surgery.

■

The price of a bypass operation varies little among Canada, Germany, and the United States—$20,000 to $30,000, depending on how complicated it is. Heart specialists the world over use identical techniques, equipment, and surgical teams. Once inside the operating room, it's virtually impossible to tell which country you are in, everything is so similar. Even the brand names of the equipment are often the same.

Yet the total heart bypass bill in the United States is far greater, because the United States does twice as many per capita. Canada and Germany both limit the number of hospitals allowed to perform bypass surgery as a way of keeping costs down. They also limit the hospitals' heart surgery budgets.

Another strategy that countries use to keep down the cost of high-technology procedures is to restrict the income of specialists who perform them. In the United States, Lankenau's Scott Goldman, with a particularly busy practice, made $700,000 before taxes in 1992. Sunnybrook's Bernard Goldman, also at the top of his profession in Canada, makes only about $280,000. Some heart surgeons in Canada make more than salaried academic physicians like Goldman. But few make much more, because the government sets physicians' fees. Reichart and other department chiefs in Germany, who bolster their salaries with privately insured patients, can do as well as top American doctors. But, on average, German heart surgeons make far less, because hospital salaries are low. They make about $80,000 a year, well below the U.S. average for heart surgeons of $296,000.

■

Most German heart-surgery patients, such as Dobler, recuperate in rehabilitation hospitals, which are more like resort hotels than hospitals. They spend a month or longer in idyllic country settings, exercising, eating healthy meals, and developing healthful lifestyles.

Typical of these facilities is the 540-bed Hoehenried Clinic, located on the shores of the Starnberger, a lovely lake about an hour's drive from Munich. With the Alps to the south and the mansions of Germany's well-to-do all about them, heart patients spend each day in the pursuit of good health.

They live in Spartan rooms with a single bed, a desk, and a picture-window view of the Starnberger and the Alps. But most of their time is spent walking on the grounds or exercising inside the low-lying modernistic facility, with its arboretums and long, glass-walled halls.

Hoehenried Clinic has a large indoor swimming pool, six gyms, a bowling alley, two biking rooms each with forty stationary bikes, and, lest anyone forget that it is a medical facility, an eight-bed intensive care unit. The staff consists of fifty doctors, thirty physiotherapists, two occupational therapists, and eight psychologists, who, among other things, conduct stress-reduction and meditation classes.

A typical day at the center begins at 7:15 A.M., with exercises on the lawns followed by breakfast. Residents return to their rooms, where they meet with their doctors for changes in their drug and exercise prescriptions. After that, they attend group discussions on healthy life-styles, followed by such exercise programs as swimming, bicycling, and rowing on the lake. In the afternoon, it's distance-walking on the wooded grounds or across rolling manicured lawns, alone or in supervised groups. Evenings are devoted to health lectures and educational and recreational movies.

Germany has fifteen centers like Hoehenried, specializing in rehabilitation for different diseases—cardiovascular, gastrointestinal, orthopedic, and neurologic. These centers are an outgrowth of the long-standing popularity of health spas in Germany, said Hubert Hofmann, medical chief at Hoehenried.

Some doctors contend that the centers are a frivolous luxury in a country with limited funds for social programs. Others argue that rehab centers ultimately save Germany money because they help restore the health of workers and return them to work.

It costs about $120 a day to stay at Hoehenried, but that doesn't bother its residents. They don't pay anything. The full cost is borne by Germany's employee pension funds.

■

While Germans revere spas and rehab centers, Americans revere technology. The U.S. health-care system promotes the use of costly technology by paying generously for the procedures without limiting their use.

Just about everyone knows that lives are being saved with kidney dialysis and kidney transplantation, that eyesight is being restored with cataract operations, that MRIs are finding brain tumors and slipped discs missed by other diagnostic methods. But few people realize how much these procedures inflate the nation's health bill.

Improved cataract surgery, made possible by advances achieved in the 1980s, costs about $3,000 per operation. It's become the most common surgical procedure on Americans over sixty-five. A total of 1.35 million Medicare recipients underwent cataract surgery in 1992—costing the government $3.4 billion. For many, the operation significantly improves eyesight and quality of life, but for others the benefits are marginal or could be had more cheaply with stronger eyeglasses.

Sometimes a new procedure is limited to a relatively small number of people but is so expensive that the total cost to society is high. The two treatments for advanced kidney disease—kidney dialysis and kidney transplantation—cost the government $6.6 billion in 1991. This is almost twice the total cost of cataract surgeries, although it benefits one-eighth as many people. Both dialysis and transplantation are financed by the federal End Stage Renal Disease Program, signed into law in 1972. Technological improvements in the treatment of this one disease have boosted the nation's health spending by almost 1 percent.

This is just one example of how technological advances increase the cost of care. A more recent high-cost procedure—bone-marrow transplantation for breast cancer—costs $150,000 per patient. Insurance companies are balking at this expense, and many are denying payment on the grounds the procedure is unproven. Should it prove worthwhile and become widespread, its cost to society would be considerable. With fifteen thousand potential candidates a year, the annual cost could come to $2.25 billion.

MRI machines came on the scene in the early 1980s. They are costing the U.S. health-care system more than $5 billion a year. The MRI is much more effective than conventional X rays in imaging joint injuries, bone-marrow disorders, soft-tissue tumors, and muscle problems, but many doctors think it's being used far too often. With a typical MRI scan costing about $1,000, they feel that cheaper diagnostic methods would be adequate in many cases.

Even very low-cost tests, if done on enough people, can greatly inflate medical expenditures. Mammograms cost about $100 each, but with 20 million American women getting these breast X rays each year, they are costing society $2 billion a year.

Few would deny that this would be money well spent if it saved many lives. But a landmark international conference by the National Cancer Institute in March 1993 concluded that mammography was frequently useless. Though it cuts deaths from breast cancer by 30 percent in women over fifty, it has little or no effect on the death rate for younger women, according to the scientists assembled by the NCI. Five million of the women who are mammographed each year in the United States are under 50. That amounts to $500 million wasted on useless tests, if the scientists are right.

Now, the American Cancer Society is promoting the use of a new, $20 test for prostate cancer, a disease that is responsible for 2 percent to 3 percent of male deaths in this country, about 35,000 deaths a year. Called PSA (prostate-specific antigen), the test has caused controversy because it fails to pick up cancer in 40 percent of cases and wrongly identifies an additional 25 percent as having the disease. Mass screening for prostate cancer, with all the follow-up care and studies to rule out the false positive tests, would cost up to $20 billion a year, says Ian M. Thompson, chief of urology at the Brooke Army Medical Center in San Antonio, who studied the matter. That would be more than 2 percent of the nation's total health bill.

In medical research, financial rewards and prestige go

to those who discover new procedures, not those who evaluate existing ones. But restricting the use of screening tests until they are clearly proved worthwhile can bring substantial savings.

The Canadian health system does pay for mammograms in older women, who do clearly benefit. But it has been saving millions every year by not giving mammograms to younger women. Canadian researchers were the first to suggest that screening younger women did not save lives. This is now gaining wide acceptance. Of course, if recent mammogram study results had gone the other way, thousands of Canadian woman might have died prematurely because their government was slow to adopt the test.

So what's a country to do?

"The high cost of medical care is reaching the point where the U.S. medical system cannot afford to provide instant gratification," said Paul Griner, president of the American College of Physicians. "The country is going to have to set priorities, hopefully priorities that won't result in terribly long queues like in Canada and Great Britain."

Harvard School of Medicine professor Howard H. Hiatt said the long-held principle of doing everything possible for the patient is a luxury society can no longer afford. "As we develop more and more practices that may be beneficial to the individual but not to the interests of society, we risk reaching a point where marginal gains to individuals threaten the welfare of the whole."

Hiatt wrote this in a controversial paper published in 1975. By 1993, he was saying that society had reached the point where its welfare was being threatened.

Says William L. Kissick, professor of health-care systems at the University of Pennsylvania's Leonard Davis Institute and author of the book *Medicine's Dilemmas: Infinite Needs vs. Finite Resources:* "No society in the world has sufficient resources to provide all the health services its population is capable of utilizing."

■

Several months after Cavallaro, Sequin, and Dobler underwent bypass surgery, each was doing fine.

Sequin was taking frequent walks in the hilly area around his home in Orillia, something he couldn't do before the surgery.

Dobler, after spending four weeks in a rehabilitation hospital, returned home to Munich and was making biking tours to keep in shape.

Cavallaro visited a cardiac rehab center near his home three times a week, to work out on a treadmill and stationary bike. He was looking forward to going to the Jersey Shore, where he would spend his summer fishing and crabbing.

CHAPTER 5

FAIRNESS: THE LAST WORD IN HEALTH-CARE REFORM

  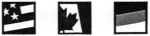

When patients in the United States seek care from a doctor or a hospital, they are immediately labeled and defined by the insurance they have. If they have Medicare, it means they're old. If they have Medicaid, it means they're poor. If they have Blue Cross or some other private insurance, it means they're probably lucky enough to have a good job and a comfortable living. Those labels are more than a notation on a file. They often determine where patients can go for care, which doctors will see them, and even the quality of care they'll get.

In Canada or Germany, a patient is just a patient. That's because, under the Canadian and German health systems, everyone is covered—and everyone is entitled to the same medical care. Two of the key components of the German and Canadian systems are equality and fairness. They are crucial, experts say, to the success of those systems.

"People have to have faith in a system for it to work," said Arthur Caplan, a medical ethicist at the University of Minnesota. "Without a set of common values there is no buy-in to a system."

In the unfolding American debate over health-care reform, the issue of fairness has been conspicuously absent. Instead, the focus is almost entirely on technical matters: Should doctors' income be capped? Should limits be placed on spending? Should drug prices be regulated? Yet economists, doctors, and health-care officials in Canada and Germany consider fairness to be inseparable from cost-effective, quality medicine.

"The experience from the industrial democracies of the world is that equal access, universal coverage, and cost controls are allies," said Alan Sager, a researcher at Boston University School of Public Health. "They are key principles used by all industrial democracies—except the United States."

As this book has shown, the United States spends more on health care than any other nation, but it leaves 37 million people uninsured. Canada and Germany both deliver quality health care to all their people, at much less cost.

They do it in different ways. Canada pays all medical bills with tax dollars. Germany covers virtually everyone through private, nonprofit insurance funds, called "sickness funds," that are highly regulated by government but funded through employer-employee contributions.

Despite their differences, both systems are grounded in the same set of principles:

- Access to health care for all.
- Equal care for all.
- Financing systems based on people's ability to pay.
- Free choice of doctors and hospitals for all.
- Limits on overall spending.

The impact of these principles on the day-to-day practice of medicine is apparent in visits to Canada and Germany, where no one asks the most common question in American medicine: "Do you have insurance?"

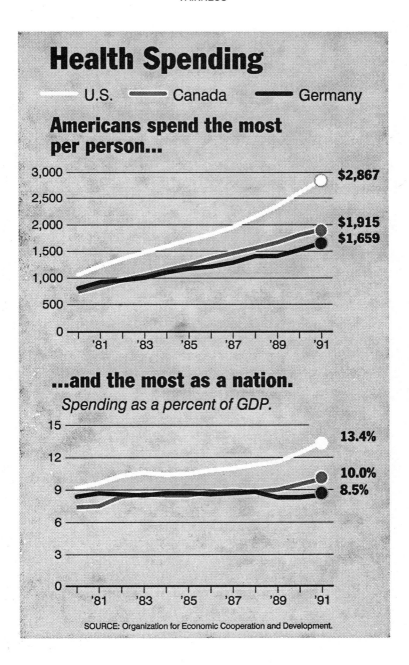

Health Spending

——— U.S.   ——— Canada   ——— Germany

Americans spend the most per person...

- 3,000 — ⚪ $2,867
- 2,500
- 2,000 — ⚫ $1,915
- 1,500 — ⚫ $1,659
- 1,000
- 500
- 0

'81 '83 '85 '87 '89 '91

...and the most as a nation.
Spending as a percent of GDP.

- 15
- ⚪ 13.4%
- 12
- ⚫ 10.0%
- 9 — ⚫ 8.5%
- 6
- 3
- 0

'81 '83 '85 '87 '89 '91

SOURCE: Organization for Economic Cooperation and Development.

Access for All

A forty-five-year-old man named Augustin was lying in the infectious-disease ward at Schwabing Hospital in Munich, talking quietly with his roommate while waiting for dinner to arrive. Augustin had a medical history that would make a U.S. insurance company shudder: He had AIDS. Yet he never worried about where he would get medical treatment, or how he would pay for it. He knew he wouldn't have to spend himself into poverty to qualify for government medical assistance, as so many Americans with catastrophic illness end up doing.

"No matter what you have, everything is paid for," said Augustin, who was getting intravenous antibiotics for pneumonia. "AIDS is no different than any other disease. There is no discrimination whatsoever."

Because health insurance isn't tied to employment status, Germans and Canadians can change jobs without worry. Switching jobs or losing a job doesn't mean losing coverage, as it often does in the United States. Augustin, for example, was still covered even though he had recently retired from his job as a psychotherapist and was living on his pension.

Dr. Dieter Eichenlaub, Schwabing's medical director and head of the hospital's AIDS program, said access for all was fundamental to the German health-care system. "We have to take everyone with everything. We can't say, 'No, we don't want you.'"

Equal Care for All

The sports medicine clinic at Toronto's North York General Hospital was filled with an assortment of athletes and injuries. On one treatment table was Adam Scott, thirteen, who had badly twisted an ankle playing basketball in the school yard. On a table across from Adam was

Bernadette Bowyer, who had torn some knee ligaments playing field hockey at the 1992 Summer Olympics in Barcelona. Both patients—the ordinary schoolboy and the Olympic athlete—were getting the same attention from the clinic's doctors and therapists.

In Canada, everyone has equal access to doctors and hospitals. There is no two-tiered system that shepherds the poor or the uninsured into public clinics while providing unlimited options for the privileged. Canadians must sometimes go on waiting lists for high-tech procedures such as heart-bypass surgery or hip replacement, but they know that no one with money or connections—or better insurance—will move ahead of them.

That same equality of treatment is basic to the German system. "It is very important to them that rich and poor people get the same health care, in the same hospitals, from the same doctors," said Uwe Reinhardt, a Princeton University health economist and an expert on the German system.

Germans with incomes above $36,000 are allowed to purchase private insurance policies. These policies give them a few extra perks, such as private hospital rooms and quicker access to some procedures. But private insurance doesn't buy anyone higher-quality care. Fewer than 10 percent of Germans choose to buy these private policies.

Fair Payment Systems

Silvana Dominelli was a construction worker's wife. Josefa Hägel was a pensioner. Peter Kessler owned a business consulting firm. Three patients, from three walks of life. All were in Schwabing Hospital, and all were getting the same level of care. Yet their insurance premiums varied widely. In Germany, what you pay depends on your ability to pay.

In 1992, the average rate for coverage under a German

Health Facts in Three Countries

Americans spend much more on health care than Germans or Canadians, but they don't live as long. Americans also see their doctors less often.

		U.S.	Canada	Germany
Health spending per capita		$2,867	$1,915	$1,659
Spending as a percent of GDP*		13.4 %	10.0 %	8.5 %
Life expectancy at birth	Women	78.8 yrs.	80.4	79.0
	Men	72.0	73.8	72.6
Doctor visits per year		5.5	6.9	10.8
Average hospital stay		9.1 days	13.9	16.5

All figures latest available, 1986=1991
SOURCE: Organization for Economic Cooperation and Development   *Gross Domestic Product

sickness fund was 12.5 percent of salary. Someone earning $40,000 would have a premium of $5,000, which would be split between the worker and the employer. For a worker earning $20,000, the premium would be just $2,500—again, shared equally by worker and employer.

Johann Fann, secretary general of the Bavarian Allgemeine Ortskrankenkasse, or AOK, Germany's largest insurance fund, said the system is based on the "social solidarity principle." "The rich pay for the poor, the young for the old, the well for the sick," he said.

In Canada, health care is financed by general tax revenues, but the end result, again, is that people who make more pay more. An average Canadian pays about 47 percent of income in taxes (compared to a total tax burden of 37 percent in the United States). In Ontario, about one-third of tax revenues goes for health care, so people earning $40,000 contribute about $6,300. People earning $20,000 would pay half that for health care.

In the United States, the cost of health care is based on how much coverage you have, not how much money you make. This puts a greater economic burden on low-wage earners.

In April 1993, the Economic Policy Institute in Washington, D.C., issued a report on how much American families spend on health care. It found that a family earning between $21,000 and $27,000 spent a larger percentage of its income on health care than a family earning between $52,000 and $72,000. When all expenses were taken into account (insurance premiums, out-of-pocket costs, and taxes to support Medicare and Medicaid), the poorer family spent 14.2 percent of its income—$3,905—on health care. The more affluent family spent only 11.4 percent of its income—$6,989—on health care. And, for its money, it got better coverage.

Freedom of Choice

Catherine Fiore, thirty-two, of Toronto, is an expert on choosing doctors and hospitals. She has bounced in and out of hospitals for about six years because of a rare viral infection of the nervous system. And she has exercised her right, under the Canadian system, to freely pick her doctor and hospital.

In fall 1992, when she grew dissatisfied with the care at Scarborough Grace Hospital, she checked out and went to North York General, seven miles away. "They were just baby-sitting me," Fiore said of Scarborough Grace. "I was looking for someone to more aggressively manage my case."

When Americans talk about reforming health care along the lines of government-run programs like Canada's, one of their main fears is losing the right to choose doctors and hospitals. That isn't a fear Canadians have. They not only can choose their doctors and hospitals, they can change their minds as often as they want if they don't like the care they're getting.

Germans, too, can go to virtually any doctor or hospital they choose.

That is more freedom than many Americans have, including the well-insured. Health maintenance organizations (HMOs), for instance, limit choices by restricting members to a pre-approved list of doctors and hospitals. Poor people's choices are limited in a different way. Even if they're on Medicaid, many doctors refuse to treat them because, they say, Medicaid fees are too low.

Overall Limits on Spending

At the end of every year, a group of doctors and insurance-fund officials gather around a conference table in a Munich office building. They are there to hammer out precisely how much Bavaria's 16,000 doctors will be paid, overall, to care for the 11 million people living in that German state. It isn't easy. The talks often go on for months.

"It is a process where we want to hold the line [financially] but ensure all care for everyone," said Johann Fann of the Bavarian AOK.

When the negotiations are concluded, the doctors walk away with a fixed sum of money from the funds. In 1991, as a result of such negotiations around the country, insurance funds handed over more than $21 billion to Germany's physicians' associations. That was all the doctors got that year—not one deutsche mark more. With that, they had to treat everyone for everything, equally. The German sickness funds also negotiate with hospitals, to decide hospital rates.

Setting fixed budgets is the single most effective cost-containment strategy used by countries such as Germany and Canada. These fixed budgets force all kinds of decisions that tend to emphasize efficiency and discourage unnecessary use of technology.

In Canada, provincial governments negotiate directly with each hospital to establish a "global budget"—a fixed amount of money the hospital must make do with for the year. The government also negotiates fee schedules and spending targets with doctors.

Because hospitals are working with a finite amount of money, doctors' incomes are kept in check, and hospitals have no incentive to give more care than needed. And because the hospitals and doctors get paid the same for all patients, they have no reason to favor a rich patient over a poor one. This removes some of the financial considerations from medical decision-making.

"While there are budgets . . . within those limits practitioners make all the clinical calls, and patients are free to choose their own doctors and hospitals," said Uwe Reinhardt of Princeton.

■

The challenge of reforming the U.S. health-care system tests the fundamental belief that, in America, anything is possible.

Up to now, people have approached medical care with the notion that there are no limits, particularly for those who can afford the best. Likewise, for the providers of health-care services—doctors, hospitals, insurance companies—the American marketplace has provided endless opportunities for financial success.

But with medical costs each year consuming a larger share of the nation's economic resources, yet leaving fewer and fewer Americans with the security of health insurance, a consensus has formed. Health care cannot go on the way it has. America now faces the difficult task of providing care to everyone, while controlling costs. While other countries have already tackled those problems, America is plunging into new territory, one that will likely involve tough choices and trade-offs.

"We still talk about health care as a market for consumption, like automobiles or refrigerators," said Deborah Stone, a professor of law and policy at Brandeis

University. "We don't have a feeling of collective responsibility." Canadians and Germans do. Europeans, said Reinhardt, "view health care as . . . part of the cement of society."

Many doubt that the United States could successfully adopt either the Canadian or German system outright. Cultural and historical differences would make that difficult. Furthermore, both the Canadian and German systems are not problem-free. Like the United States, those countries are struggling with the rising costs of technology and the need to care for burgeoning numbers of elderly people. Their citizens, too, demand the latest in modern medicine.

All ten of Canada's provinces are reeling from health-care inflation, and they are imposing sharp budgetary restrictions on medical care. Eight times between 1977 and 1989, Germany made significant changes to restrain spending.

But looking at both these systems is useful. It can help guide U.S. policy-makers as they move through the process of revamping health care. And it can help all Americans find the right questions to ask:

Will health insurance cover everyone?

Will everyone get equal care?

Will the financial burden be equitably shared?

Will overall spending be limited?

In the end, will the health care system be fair?